Medicine in America
Historical Essays

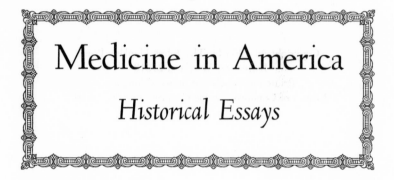

Medicine in America

Historical Essays

Richard Harrison Shryock

The Johns Hopkins Press
Baltimore, Maryland

To Owsei Temkin—
colleague and friend

Foreword

Having long appreciated the pioneer contributions of Professor Shryock to the history of the medical sciences, the development of the medical profession, the public health movement, and the relation of all these to the social and intellectual history of the United States I know that these essays, selected from a large body of his scattered writings, are sure to be welcomed by specialists who will find it convenient to have them assembled in a single, accessible volume. The essays speak so cogently for themselves that any comment or "introduction" seems needless and even gratuitous. But perhaps I can point out a few of the significant characteristics of these essays for the general student of American cultural history who, in the vast and rapid proliferation of specialized studies in the field may not have a first-hand acquaintance with them. Such a student has before him a rich intellectual experience.

All the essays reflect one of the notable contributions of Professor Shryock to American historiography. He not only chose an almost completely ignored chapter in the national history; he also described and analyzed medical, scientific, and public health developments within a large and meaningful context. The essays, in terms of the time they were written, show that he was one of the first historians to report and evaluate an American story within the knowledgeable frame of western thought from the Greeks to our own time. In explaining American developments in relation to trans-Atlantic civilization he has not only shown the indebtedness of Americans to Europe; he has also shown the originality of many of the American developments themselves. No less important has been the clear and precise way in which American interest in medicine and public health has been related to major American historical processes: to plantation life and slavery, with new light on the debate on the treatment or mistreatment of slaves; to urbanism, with a fresh understanding of the contributions of medical men to the deleterious effects on city life and to the impact of this concern on the growth of civic responsibility and social control; to democracy, with the complex interrelations between folk traditions, assumptions, and prejudices and tested knowledge and sophisticated skills; to the shifting status, role, interests and opportunities of women, with convincing answers to the question why America pioneered in many ways in opening medical training and practice to women; and to war, particularly the Civil War. From his analyses and insight every student of these major historical experiences can derive larger and deeper understanding.

Whatever his field of special interest the practitioner and student of American history can learn a good deal from the ways Professor Shryock has handled historical problems. His approach has been exploratory; he has brought to the foreground important but neglected problems and issues. It has been both expository and analytical. His balanced judgments reflect the best canons of scholarship and show shrewd insight and controlled imagination in approaching and dealing with specific historical questions. On re-reading the essays I am struck by the fact that long before the currently fashionable concern of many younger historians with the methods and concepts of the behavioral sciences, Professor Shryock was fully aware of variables and their control and of the critical and fruitful use of statistical procedures. These methods, evident in so many of the essays, are particularly striking in the celebrated answer he has given to the question why Americans lagged in basic scientific research. These qualities also inform his exposition of the reasons why the Anglo-American physician William Charles Wells, anticipating Darwin in a paper written in 1813, failed to have the influence on later developments in evolutionary theory that might be expected. I do not know a more significant methodological contribution to American intellectual history than the one in this essay. Professor Shryock brilliantly unravels the bearings on the "discovery" of a theory and its "influence" on *both* the internal analysis and exposition of the discoverer's observation and insight, on the one hand, and the social and cultural situation and milieu on the other.

Without straining for relevances, Professor Shryock often gives us light on the implications of earlier developments, on issues of our own day. This appears in many of the essays. It is especially noteworthy in "The Historical Significance of the Tuberculosis Movement" and in the essays comparing the medical situation "then and now." Also relevant to our own times are his contributions to an understanding of such topics as specialization and psychosomatic medicine, the support and control of research by voluntary and state agencies, the struggle for professional standards in the context of competition, desire for profits and prestige, and humanitarian values.

The reader of these essays, interested in method, will also be struck by Professor Shryock's broadened recognition of pertinent sources. He has made excellent use of medical journals and reports, diaries and correspondence, and newspaper accounts. In his analyses of travel accounts and of statistics he has given us examples of new uses of familiar sources of historical information. One example of a fruitful use of Tocqueville's unsatisfactory explanation of the American emphasis on the "utilitarian" as opposed to the "theoretical" is evidenced in the careful definition of the operative terms together with such words as "business man," "middle class," and "the multitude."

These essays are also models of clear exposition of technical material. The reader will also appreciate the skillful use of "human interest" in connection with men who have suffered in "the conflict with oblivion." Finally the wit and urbanity of the writing, especially in handling professional quarrels and popular prejudices, adds a delightful component to this book.

University of Wisconsin   MERLE CURTI

Preface

Most families consult lawyers only at rare intervals. Children see teachers regularly, but chiefly in groups as a matter of routine; while many persons have no contact with clergymen from one year to the next. But it is an unusual family which does not call for the services of a doctor, a dentist, or some other health specialist at least once a year—often as a personal matter thought to be critical in nature. This dependence on medical personnel, moreover, is increasing: in 1930, the average American made about 2.5 visits to a physician annually; by 1960 this figure had risen to 5.3. Similar statements could be made about a growing resort to clinics, hospitals, and so-called nursing homes. All these facts indicate confidence in medical services, and opinion polls have placed physicians at the top of the professions. "Dr. Kildare" and various other "TV" programs, "comics," and "movies" have pictured hospitals as dramatic and even glamorous institutions. In view of this esteem and the growing desire for medical care, many plans have been made to help families meet the mounting costs of such care—particularly through health insurance of a voluntary or compulsory nature.

Yet, paradoxically, there is, and has long been, considerable distrust of the medical profession. Americans are still said to be suspicious of physicians in general, although devoted to their own doctors in particular. Doubts have been further aroused as demands for compulsory health insurance have been opposed by "organized medicine." When the federal "medicare" law finally provided hospital services for elderly people, this added to the anxieties of the public at large. For they now worried about the quantity as well as the quality of medical service. Unfortunately, the ratio of doctors to patients fell between 1910 and 1940, since better standards of training reduced medical graduates just when population expansion accelerated. It has been apparent for two decades that there were not enough doctors or nurses to meet American expectations, and "medicare" will require even more such personnel the moment it goes into operation in 1966.

Most persons now desire more as well as better doctors and nurses, but to train such personnel is a slow and costly process. It is estimated that after an investment of from five to ten years in planning, and of at least $30 million, a single medical school can be founded, but will then provide only one hundred new doctors a year. Yet recruits for the medical, and related, guilds will be needed in the tens of thousands within another decade. No wonder that *Harpers Magazine* ran a series of articles several years ago entitled "The Crisis in American Medicine."

There have been crises in medicine before; indeed, this has been almost the normal state of things since medical science began to stir from its ancient lethargy some three centuries ago. For one reason or another, however, difficulties in this field seem to become more serious in terms of public consciousness if not of actual needs.

In any case, historians should not make the mistake of viewing this medical story as a highly specialized one merely tangential to general history. Nor should they commit the lesser, but still serious, error of viewing it as only one chapter in the history of science. In some respects, of course, medical history does overlap and even coincides with that of science.

Yet medicine, as is always noted, is more than science: it is also an art. Moreover, because it deals with the vital interests of both individuals and societies—with life and death, and with so much that matters in between—medicine has long had an unusually complex and intimate relationship to social and cultural developments at large. Hence the term "medical history," as here employed, is broad indeed, involving the history of disease and of all attempts—magical or scientific, biologic or social—to promote health and to prevent, cure, or ameliorate illness. It follows that the concept includes past trends in "social medicine" (the mutual interaction of social conditions and disease) and in "medical sociology" (interrelations of medical institutions and personnel, forms and costs of medical care, and so on). In other words, medical history involves social and economic as well as biologic content and presents one of the central themes in human experience. After all, what is more basic in the life of any people than life itself?

The need to preserve or restore health has been obvious in all societies, even as has the need to train the young (educational history), or the necessity of maintaining order and assuring co-operation (political and legal history). The relatively technical aspects of medicine, as of law—which likewise has long combined specialized learning with human concerns —seem to have disinclined historians from giving these fields adequate attention. But just to the extent that this is true, the resulting narratives are incomplete and at times misleading.

American medical history can be conveniently divided into certain chronologic periods. Theoretically, any one of its various aspects would provide a criterion for this purpose; for example, the state of public health, or the nature of medical care. Such themes, however are external to medical science proper, which evolves partly by virtue of its own internal logic —as when discovery "b" can be made only after discovery "a" regardless of time, place, or circumstance. It is this story of science and related practice which presents the most distinctive aspect of medical history and therefore offers the most useful guide for periodization.

When this criterion is used, there emerge five eras which provide meaningful contrasts, but which rarely correspond to the periods employed by political or economic historians. These eras, arbitrary in terms of exact dates, may be defined as (1) Early Colonial, 1620–1720: Quasi-medieval thought and crude empiricism; (2) The Second Century, 1720–1820: Speculative "systems" of pathology and heroic practice; (3) The Middle Period, 1820–1870: Advent of "modern" pathology and clinical studies; (4) The Germanic Epoch, 1870–1920: Early influence of science on public health and surgery; and (5) The Recent Era, 1920–1965: Acceleration of medical progress.

Students of American history, or of American studies, may find it difficult to reconcile these categories with conventional time divisions set by presidential administrations, major wars, industrial revolutions, and so on. There are, of course, some overlappings. Thus, the third era noted above corresponds roughly to what often *has* been termed the "Middle Period" of American history. And since there is a continuing interplay between external influences (cultural factors) and the internal logic of medicine, it is helpful to know one tradition in relation to another. "Jacksonian democracy," industrial developments following 1850, and various other social trends had their implications for both science and practice.

On the other hand, the space divisions (regions or "sections") so emphasized in general history have less significance for medicine. Most differences which did appear between disease patterns and medical practice in one area and in another were minor ones, although such contrasts were at times exaggerated for political purposes. (At present, the only major phenomenon is the inadequacy of medical care in rural areas in all parts of the country—a type of regionalism rarely stressed by general historians.) Perhaps it was this lack of sectional emphasis which made it so easy to reunite the medical profession after 1865, in comparison to the schisms which long persisted within the Protestant churches and to a lesser degree within political parties and other bodies.

Only one of the chapters in this volume ("Medical Practice in the Old South") is limited to a particular region—to the area which actually was most distinctive in this context. Several of the chapters relate to only one epoch (1820–1870), such as those concerning indifference to basic science, the origins of the public health movement, and the Civil War. Two focus on the thought of individuals; namely, of the forgotten New Englander Sylvester Graham (of Graham crackers fame); and of the almost-forgotten Charlestonian William Charles Wells, whose scientific contributions far outranked those of any other American physician of his era (1790–1815). With the exception of this essay on Wells (who was as much English as American), and of one other, all the chapters relate primarily to the history of this country.

Two chapters—the brief statement on studies in the history of American science, and that on the public health, mentioned above—are included as early examples of a professional interest maintained in this field over the past forty years. Both of these items are now "dated" by subsequent, more comprehensive studies on similar themes. Except in these cases, however, all materials selected are chosen in the belief that their content is pertinent to present scholarship.

Various papers, although appropriate in subject matter, have been omitted in order to avoid excessive length. Such caution is essential for an author convinced that his type of work, if it is to avoid distortion, must be largely impersonal, rarely dramatic, and never glamorous. This being so, he cannot expect that many persons will ever read all that he has written. Yet even those who are chiefly concerned with other aspects of national experience may still wish to know something of the medical factors in that experience. It is for such readers that the first chapter in the present volume has been prepared, as a summarized version of American medical history as a whole.

This résumé is also indicated, as medical men would say, by the persisting lack of any full-length treatment of the subject. Lest this statement be misunderstood, I hasten to express my admiration for and indebtedness to the pioneer volumes by Dr. Francis R. Packard, and to the shorter work by Dr. Henry E. Sigerist on American medicine. But for various reasons, neither of these contributions—valuable as they are—supplies the synthesis now needed by professional historians and perhaps by social scientists as well. Neither, for that matter, can the introductory chapter fully serve this end, but it may provide a step in that direction. Although little can be claimed for the essay's "research design," one may at least muster up enough courage to term it a "pilot study."

It is hoped, at the same time, that those who have succumbed to the lure of medical history as such will find it convenient to have these materials brought together (from a dozen journals, dated between 1930 and 1962) into a single volume. At first glance, the collection may seem a potpourri, but actually it is arranged in terms of such inherent categories as medical science, the medical professions, historiography, and so on. Viewed separately, certain chapters may interest only certain readers; taken together, the whole is—hopefully—more than the sum of its parts. Here, at least, are some of the elements, and possibly some of the interpretations, which will enter into the more complete synthesis of the future.

The American Philosophical Society
Philadelphia, 1966   RICHARD HARRISON SHRYOCK

Contents

THE MEDICAL PROFESSION

MEDICAL THOUGHT AND RESEARCH

HISTORIOGRAPHY

Medicine in America
Historical Essays

I

The Medical History
of the American People

Illness among the American Indians, both before and long
after the arrival of the first Europeans, was combated by
medical practices which combined magic and empiricism in
varying degrees. Futile as most of this practice must have
been, modern observers credit "white magic" with some
psychosomatic value, and the partial success of native empiricism is attested by the number of native drugs which found
their way into European pharmacopoeias. Most of these were
simply emetics or cathartics (such as jalap, or the present
cascara), but one—Inca cinchona bark—proved to be the first
truly "specific" drug discovered and exerted influence on
European medical theory as well as on practice. Fortunately
for the Indians, moreover, they seem to have been unafflicted
originally by some of the most serious European and African
plagues.

The "coming of the white man," and of the "black" as well,
suddenly exposed the natives to diseases against which they
had acquired no immunity; though it is an old cliché—not
fully substantiated—that the indigenes repaid in kind by
spreading syphilis among the invaders. America certainly
became a melting pot of diseases as well as of peoples, as
Indians, Europeans, and Negroes engaged in a free exchange

of their respective infections. The former suffered the most in this process, and many of the small tribes of the Caribbean and of the eastern seaboard of the future United States seem to have been almost wiped out by this biologic warfare. Although usually unplanned, the outcome was viewed with some equanimity by many English leaders. In 1702, for example, the Rev. Cotton Mather of Boston made his famous (or infamous) statement, that as a result of epidemics "the woods were almost cleared of those pernicious creatures, to make room for a better growth." [1]

The whites themselves did not fare too well during the first century of colonization. Long remembered was the terrible winter of sickness at Plymouth and "the starving time" in Virginia. Without continued immigration, the latter settlement would have died out—partly because of the lack of women, but also as a result of disease.[2] Winter mortality was caused chiefly by the usual respiratory diseases and by malnutrition (scurvy, possibly pellagra); summer deaths resulted from gastro-enteritis and malaria. When, as in the last named entity, insect vectors were involved, it required some time before human carriers could infect the innocent mosquito population. Hence, in most instances, early settlements were joyfully reported most "salubrious," but subsequently were devastated by both endemic and epidemic "fevers." Among the latter, the most feared outbreaks were those of "throat distemper" (diphtheria) and of smallpox. During the first century the isolation of small villages provided some protection against contagion. Hence smallpox, endemic in England, appeared only sporadically in epidemic form. But such protec-

[1] In his *Magnalia Christi Americana*, I, Hartford, 1855 (original ed. 1702), 51. On the total effects on Indian peoples, see P. M. Ashburn, *Ranks of Death*, New York, 1947, *passim*.

[2] See, e.g., W. Blanton, "Epidemics, Real and Imaginary, and Other Factors Influencing Seventeenth Century Virginia's Population," *Bull. Med. Hist.*, XXXI, 1957, 454–62.

tion declined with the extension of settlements and with improvements in transportation.[3]

Endemic conditions, though taken for granted and thus less alarming, always caused the most deaths. Chief among them were malnutrition, malaria, and possibly tuberculosis. There is no reason to doubt that degenerative and malignant diseases were common among the elderly, but so small a proportion of the population survived to an advanced age that these illnesses aroused no general concern. The death rate, by modern standards, was very high but was more than balanced by a maximum birth rate. Since infections were most fatal among small children, life expectancy at birth was low (about twenty-five to thirty years?), and the percentage of children in the total population was correspondingly high.[4] Natural increase in population was relatively slow.

Death was so frequent an experience within families that its inevitability and religious implications were impressed even upon small children. It is difficult to say how far this attitude reflected prevailing Calvinism, and how far it was an effort to make a virtue of necessity. Only rarely was there a note of protest; as when Cotton Mather—lamenting infant mortality in 1720—exclaimed: [5]

O how unsearchable the Judgements of God, and His Ways past finding out! The lamps but just litt up, and blown out again.

[3] On Colonial epidemics at large, see J. Duffy, *Epidemics in Colonial America*, Baton Rouge, La., 1953. The most thorough study of endemic infection, is St. Julien R. Childs, *Malaria and Colonization in the Carolina Low Country, 1526–1696*, Baltimore, 1940.

[4] There are practically no vital statistics for the seventeenth century, though the fragmentary evidence of family bibles, tombstones, diaries, etc., usually points in the directions noted. It has been roughly estimated that half of all children died before the age of ten. But cf. T. J. Wertenbaker, *The First Americans: 1607–1690*, New York, 1938, pp. 181–86.

[5] O. T. Beall, Jr. and R. H. Shryock, *Cotton Mather: First Significant Figure in American Medicine*, Baltimore, 1954, p. 76.

The very fact that population patterns were similar to those observed until recently in "undeveloped" countries, implies that medical resources were most limited. Although progress in anatomy promised some aid to surgery and obstetrics by the 1600's, and both experiments and quantitative methods were then beginning to be applied in physiology, these advances in European science exerted little influence on medical practice on either side of the Atlantic. Medical thought continued to focus on the general state of patients' "systems," which was usually explained by classical assumptions anent the state of body fluids (humors)—blood, bile, and phlegm, especially the former.

Hence, cures were sought through depletion procedures (bleeding, purging, and so on) which would rid the body of excess or impure fluids, transfusions which would overcome a lack of blood (soon abandoned because dangerous), and the use of a complex list of drugs supposed to achieve similar results. Surgery, despite greater anatomic knowledge and a few technical improvements, was limited to such structural emergencies as fractures, amputations, and occasional "cutting for stone." Surgeons also took care of skin conditions, but played no role in internal medicine. Where was the man who could operate on impure blood?

Even the English physician Sydenham, who decided that patients suffered from distinct entities rather than just from generalized, humoral states, still held that these "specific" diseases (identified and diagnosed by symptoms) could be treated only by the same methods as have been mentioned. Diseases with striking, superficial symptoms had long been vaguely distinguished: hence, such names as great pox (syphilis), small pox, yellow fever, scarlet fever, and so on. But for most medical men, distinctions between entities were largely academic, since they had little bearing on treatments. Practitioners differed chiefly on such matters as when, where, how often, and how extensively bleeding should be pursued, or what regimen or what particular drugs were to be employed.

A sensible "doctor" could of course provide moral support, but this was not likely to lower mortality rates. Nor were the traditional, preventive practices—isolation and sanitation—well enough understood or applied to attain this same end. / The most that can be claimed for the medical practice of the period was (1) moral or psychosomatic values, (2) minor amelioration (as in the use of opiates), (3) the handling of structural emergencies, and (4) occasional checks to contagion by severe quarantine regulations.[6] /

Under these circumstances, a prompt exportation of the best English medical facilities to the Colonies would have provided only minor aid. Yet even this was long denied to the overseas provinces. Isolation and poverty explain neglect in part, especially during the earliest decades; but policy—or rather the lack of it—was also responsible. Unlike the Spanish, the English (and later the British) government made no effort to project a medical code overseas. Such matters as the licensing of practitioners, medical ethics, medical costs, and so on, were left to the provinces themselves—a tradition later inherited by the states in the Union.

Meantime, ~~neither~~ the Anglican Church nor non-conformist bodies maintained the medieval tradition of caring for the sick poor, and no nursing orders survived which might have assumed this function. The English government, ~~moreover~~, failed to move into the resulting welfare vacuum, leaving the maintenance of both hospitals and medical education to voluntary initiative./ Such initiative gradually took form in

[6] Accounts of the medical thought and practice of the period are available in all general texts. A brief discussion is given in R. H. Shryock, *Medicine and Society in America*, New York, 1960, pp. 47–51. See also L. S. King, *The Medical World of the Eighteenth Century*, Chicago, 1958, *passim*.

London and a few other large towns in Britain, but was lacking in colonial villages. Hence the Colonies long possessed no medical schools, societies, or hospitals. Most routine care was based on folk medicine, including that secured at times from the Indians. Even men termed "doctors" did not hesitate to seek help where they could find it. The favorite remedies of the Rev. Gershow Bulkeley were borrowed from a Hartford blacksmith.[7]

Although concern about licensing practitioners was occasionally expressed in legislatures, no control was possible in the absence of formal education. Both men and women engaged in medical practice at will, often combining it with other pursuits. They usually charged fees for service. A few such persons were graduates of arts colleges founded before 1720, and here and there men with some European training were available.

Certain of the best medical men were clergymen, since both their education and ideals were usually superior; and this persistence of clerical practice was still common in England as well as in the American provinces. But, at best, most practitioners were trained only by apprenticeship. All of them were termed "doctors," but in effect they resembled the surgeon-apothecaries of rural Britain—engaging necessarily in surgery and drug-selling as well as general practice. Only after 1720 did increasing wealth enable a few Americans to secure formal education abroad, and so to return home as "physicians" in the London sense; that is, as elite practitioners with university backgrounds.[8]

Summing up the first-century story, one may say that disease conditions in America were, if anything, even more serious than in Europe; that European medical science,

[7] W. R. Steiner, "The Rev. Gershow Bulkely . . . ," *Johns Hopkins Hosp. Bull.*, XVII, 1906, 48 ff.

[8] Shryock, n. 6 above, pp. 2–15.

inadequate as it was, reached the Colonies to only a limited degree, and that death rates were appalling. Medical care was largely ignored by both Church and State, and voluntary medical services—uncontrolled and usually of dubious quality—reflected an unplanned adjustment of British traditions to the American scene. Thus society molded medical care in many ways, but little reverse influence on society can be observed.

Despite technical advances in medical practice during the later eighteenth century, as in the work of the Hunters in London in surgery and obstetrics, this was a confused period in medical thought. Newtonian triumphs inspired a hope that the physical sciences could be applied systematically to the solution of medical problems. But this belief, though prophetic, was premature at the time. Disillusionment led some physicians to react against all "rational" approaches, and to focus simply on a trial-and-error search for remedies. Such empiricism occasionally "paid off," as in Dr. Withering's discovery of the drug digitalis; or, notably, in another borrowing from folk medicine in the case of the introduction of inoculation against smallpox.

Here was the advent of a strictly "preventive" medicine, and its first large-scale, successful use was directed by Cotton Mather and Dr. Boylston in the Boston epidemic of 1721. By employing a simple calculus of probability—itself a pioneer use of quantification in medicine—they demonstrated that smallpox case mortality dropped from about 15 per cent ("in the natural way") to 1 or 2 per cent after inoculation with the disease "virus." The Boston demonstration encouraged considerable use of the process in England after 1730 and on the Continent after 1750. Jenner's "vaccination" of 1799, although much safer and more effective, was in principle a

modification of the earlier inoculation procedure. The
Mather-Boylston achievement may be viewed as the chief
American contribution to medicine prior to the mid-nine-
teenth century.[9]

Also promising was a slowly growing interest in Sydenham's concept of specific diseases, which resulted in better
descriptions of "clinical pictures." But since such identifica-
tions were still based on symptoms alone, "rational" doctors
were tempted to classify all known symptomatic entities in
systems of "nosology." This approach proved successful when
the Swedish physician Linnaeus applied it to botanic taxonomy, but led to endless confusion in medicine when hundreds
of names for symptom-complexes were listed as separate
diseases. Again disillusioned, some medical leaders went to the
other extreme of repudiating "specificity" altogether, and
continued to emphasize only general states of the body. The
majority retained the traditional humoral concept and its
related depletion therapy.

Meantime, another Greek concept was revived; namely,
that illness was primarily a general state of the nervous and
vascular systems ("solidism"), and that therapy should be
devoted to either quieting tension in these parts, or to
stimulating them when they exhibited a lack of tone.[10] This
view migrated from German and Dutch schools to Edinburgh,
and young Americans took it over while studying in the latter
city. Benjamin Rush, in particular, carried the theory to
extremes after returning to Philadelphia. All illness, he held,
resulted from tension in the blood vessels; and all could be

[9] Note 5 above, Chapters 4 and 5; Genevieve Miller, *The Adoption of
Inoculation for Smallpox in England and France,* Phila., 1957, pp.
109 ff.

[10] On the development of pathology and therapy in this era, see especially
Knud Faber, *Nosography,* 2 ed., New York, 1930; E. R. Long, *History of
Pathology,* Baltimore, 1928; and the contemporary American essays by D.
Ramsay (1801) and by Edward Miller (1803).

cured by the bleeding and purging which relaxed these vessels. He seemed to prove his point; anyone could see that a patient—if bled long enough—*would* "relax" sooner or later! Rush's popularity as a writer and teacher spread the blight of heroic practice across the United States for half a century, 1800–1850. Prior to that era, bleeding had been moderate in terms of the alternative, humoral pathology.[11]

Somewhat paradoxically, this spread of Rush's "system" was made possible by progress in the organizing of a medical profession and of medical institutions. Almshouses, on the English model, appeared in Boston in 1685, and in Philadelphia in 1732, and both set up infirmaries which evolved into primitive hospitals. In the latter city Quaker influence aided Dr. Thomas Bond in founding the first hospital in the modern sense (The Pennsylvania Hospital) in the early 1750's. This institution, and the New York Hospital established just before the Revolution, followed British examples in their "voluntary" pattern; that is, they depended largely upon private funds and were governed by lay trustees. Hospitals, like the early arts colleges, thus maintained the English tradition, in contrast to the Continental tendency to place such bodies under the control of Church or State.[12]

Several medical societies were founded in the larger towns between 1730 and 1770, as practice became more profitable and young doctors with European training began to provide

[11] For recent interpretations of Rush's medical thought, see appendix to G. W. Corner, ed., *Autobiography of Benjamin Rush,* Princeton, 1948; and Shryock, "Benjamin Rush from the Perspective of the Twentieth Century," *Trans.,* College of Physicians of Phila., 4 ser., XIV, Dec., 1946, 113–20.

[12] The Pennsylvania Hospital has preserved its archives for more than two centuries, and microfilm copies up to about 1860 are available in the Library of the American Philosophical Society. On the early almshouses, see Carl Bridenbaugh, *Cities in the Wilderness,* New York, 1938, pp. 81, 394; and R. J. Hunter, "Benjamin Franklin and the Rise of Free Treatment of the Poor by the Medical Profession of Philadelphia," *Bull. Med. Hist.,* XXX, 1957, 142–44.

leadership. In 1765 Dr. John Morgan founded the first American medical school (or first British provincial school?) in Philadelphia. This was modeled on Edinburgh in being associated with an arts faculty (the College of Philadelphia). Hence, it maintained the general European tradition of locating medical education in universities, rather than the peculiar English arrangement of providing such training within London hospitals. A similar medical school was founded at King's College shortly thereafter, and at Harvard College in the 1780's.[13]

The existence of native medical schools made more acute the old problem of standardizing practice by licensing procedures. The local medical societies, and the first provincial society (New Jersey, 1761), all wished to distinguish between the better-grade practitioners and those with little or no training even by apprenticeship. Dr. Morgan hoped to go further by setting up in Philadelphia a replica of the College of Physicians of London, which would license (for all the Colonies) only men holding medical degrees—true physicians in the London sense. These leaders would eschew surgery and drug-selling.[14] Distinctions between such men and surgeons or apothecaries, however, were not feasible in provincial towns on either side of the Atlantic. Actually, the American who held a medical degree enjoyed prestige, but engaged in all types of practice just as did men who lacked formal training.

About 1760 New York set up the first examining and licensing program, although this applied only to New York City. Then, in 1772, the New Jersey Society persuaded the Legislature to provide an Examining Board and licensure for the entire province—with penalties for violations. (This pioneer law was signed by Governor William Franklin, son of

---

[13] Eventually, the College of Philadelphia became the University of Pennsylvania; and King's College, Columbia University.

[14] W. J. Bell, Jr., *John Morgan*, Phila., 1965, Chapters 7 and 8.

Benjamin Franklin.) [15] The outbreak of the Revolution in 1776 delayed further legislation of this sort; but military needs brought many "doctors" together from different states, and commanders felt it necessary to test unknown candidates for the medical services. Many "doctors" thus became familiar with examining procedures, and this doubtless encouraged them to urge licensing arrangements in their respective states at the end of the War.[16] Between 1780 and 1810 most states responded; placing licensure in some cases in the hands of state-appointed boards (as in New Jersey), or else assigning this function to the state medical societies founded during the same era (as in Massachusetts).

In the latter case, however, a controversy arose as to whether men who passed "exams" at the new Harvard Medical School should also have to take those set by the medical society. The outcome was an arrangement by which either a recognized medical degree or the passage of the state society's tests qualified a man for practice.[17] In permitting both schools and societies to license graduates, Massachusetts was following the English example of allowing the universities, as well as the societies (the old medical corporations) to extend licensing privileges. Most American states, likewise, extended such authority to medical schools after about 1820. From the beginning, however, American licensure was usually intended to limit rights to approved candidates (hence, penalties for unauthorized practice), whereas English laws only prohibited misrepresentation of a "doctor's" qualifications.[18] This distinc-

---

[15] On the New York Law, see *The New York Gazette*, June 16, 1760; on the New Jersey act, S. Allison, ed., *Acts of the General Assembly of the Province of New Jersey, 1702–1776* (XII George III), Burlington, N.J., 1776.

[16] B. Hindle, *The Pursuit of Science in Revolutionary America, 1735–1789*, Chapel Hill, North Carolina, 1956, p. 236.

[17] Josiah Bartlett, . . . *Progress of Medical Science in . . . Massachusetts*, Boston, 1810, pp. 15–25.

[18] Cf. F. N. L. Poynter, "The Influence of Government Legislation on Medical Practice in Britain," in Poynter, ed., *Evolution of Medical*

tion has been maintained throughout the history of the two countries, although one might have expected these positions to have been reversed.

Thus, by 1800, American society had established medical institutions totally lacking a half-century earlier—medical societies, schools, hospitals, and licensure. These accomplishments, reflecting growing population and wealth, British influences, and the spirit of the Enlightenment, would alone have made for professional pride. Combined with the enthusiasm engendered by a successful revolution, the outcome by 1820 was a state of mind bordering on euphoria. Within the memory of older doctors American medicine had progressed from a state of colonial dependence and mediocrity to a level which (they claimed) invited favorable comparisons with the Old World.[19]

It was true that infectious diseases continued to devastate the country, as in the terrible epidemics of yellow fever in port cities between 1790 and 1825; but there were premonitions of improvement in the public health in various respects. The use of cinchona bark (after about 1720) gave some control over malaria, and vaccination did the same for small pox. In New England, indeed, malaria practically disappeared. The first statistical estimates (for the later eighteenth century) indicated a life expectancy at birth of only thirty-five years, but certain able doctors thought they could recall signs of a declining infant mortality rate.[20] Certain other diseases, moreover—scurvy and bubonic plague—seemed to be declining. So encouraging was all this that Benjamin Franklin, as well as

Practice in Britain, London, 1961, pp. 5–15; and B. Spector, "The Growth of Medicine and the Letter of the Law," *Bull. Hist. Med.*, vol. 26, Nov., 1962, pp. 499–525.

[19] See, e.g., N. Chapman, *Phila. Jour. Med. and Physical Science*, I, 1820, 9.

[20] David Ramsay, *A Review of the Improvements, Progress and State of Medicine in the XVIIIth Century*, Charleston, S.C., 1801, p. 26.

certain French *philosophes,* envisaged a future when men would live to an indefinite age.[21]

The "Middle Period" of American medicine, 1820–1870, seems disillusioning in that it opened at a time of optimism, only to encounter subsequent frustration and confusion. In 1765 John Morgan had predicted the appearance of true physicians; yet in the 1840's, doctors were lamenting the "declining state" of their profession. In 1789 Dr. Rush had announced that his system of practice was more perfect "than the world had yet seen"; yet half a century later his views and practice were ridiculed within his own guild. Thus, Oliver Wendell Holmes remarked of Rush that he:

> . . . could not help feeling as if Nature had been a good deal shaken by the Declaration of Independence, and that American art was getting to be rather too much for her— especially as illustrated in his own practice.[22]

Finally, and most seriously, Dr. Ramsay had estimated in 1801 that health conditions were improving, but within another generation it appeared that mortality rates in American cities were rising ominously.[23]

Considering first the disease trends of this era, degenerative or malignant conditions presumably remained constant. If there were ups or downs in such morbidity there are no reliable indications. This is partly because good statistical studies were only getting under way in the 1850's, partly

[21] Franklin to Joseph Priestley, Passy, France, 1780, in W. T. Franklin, ed., *Private Correspondence of Benjamin Franklin,* 2 ed., London, I, 1817, 52; A. Deutsch, *The Mentally Ill in America,* New York, 1946, Chapters 2–6.

[22] Holmes, "Currents and Counter-Currents in Medical Science" (1860), in his collected papers of the same title, Cambridge, Mass., 1861, pp. 11 and 26 f.

[23] Shryock, *Medicine and Society in America: 1660–1860,* pp. 117 f.

because some of the disease entities were not yet recognized and so could not be enumerated in any case. A slight rise by 1850 in life expectancy at birth brought the average to almost forty years, but this would not have so increased the elderly population element as to influence mortality from the conditions mentioned.

Indeed, the saving of lives was largely limited to those of children, while young and middle-aged persons suffered as before from infectious diseases. In view of the continued ineffectiveness of both therapy and public health measures, moreover, such increase as occurred in life expectancy can be largely ascribed to a slow rise in living standards rather than to medical measures. Better standards were made possible by potential resources now becoming actual at the touch of technology, as well as by such other factors as immigrant labor, and the geographical isolation which made military service and expenditures unnecessary.[24]

The urban poor, of course, benefited little if any from increased productivity, particularly in a laissez faire era when they received no state aid save in emergencies. At the same time, they were exposed to slum conditions which seem to have been more dangerous than those confronted in rural areas.[25] These facts probably explain the increasing death rates reported in large cities, between 1825 and 1850.

Broken down into disease entities, the chief endemic infections continued to be enteritis in summer and respiratory conditions in winter. Malaria, although largely eliminated

[24] E. W. Martin, *The Standard of Living in 1860*, Chicago, pp. 220, 393–404.

[25] Although conditions in contemporary English slums were also appalling, as revealed in Chadwick's famous survey of 1842, recent British studies have suggested that the standards of even the "labouring classes" were rising slowly, 1820–1850. But read the work by J. H. Griscom, *Sanitary Condition of the Laboring Population of New York . . .* , New York, 1845; or the reports of the Committee on Hygiene of the A.M.A., 1847–1850, in the *Trans.* of that body, for the American picture.

from New England and the Middle Atlantic states, remained
a major plague in the Middle West as well as in the South.[26]
There is some evidence that malnutritional diseases, declining
in the North because of better living conditions, persisted
among the poorer classes (including the slaves) in the South.
But "the captain of the men of death" by 1850 was clearly
"consumption" (largely pulmonary tuberculosis); and if statistics were available, they might show that this had already
been true during the preceding century. Smallpox, although
under some control, remained one of the chief causes of death
in cities as late as 1860 (through neglect of vaccination).
Unrecognized, and not fatal but still serious, was hookworm
infection in the South. Just how fatal medical practice itself
was, we do not know, since therapy was never listed among
the causes of death.

The most alarming epidemic diseases of the era were yellow
fever, limited to the South after 1825, and the cholera which
so alarmed the nation in the 1830's, the '40's, and the '60's.[27] It
was these two entities whose natures were best calculated to
arouse terror, and which therefore inspired public health
measures to a greater degree than did the more devastating
tuberculosis. The latter infection was even romanticized, as in
the case of genteel females "going into a decline," and so made
a morbid contribution to art and letters.[28]

Paradoxically, this era when death rates remained high, was
at the same time a most promising epoch in medical science.
As early as 1760, when physicians described morbid as well as
normal anatomy, the Italian, Morgagni, had made clear a
means for ending the confusion in medical taxonomy. If
diseases were identified not simply by symptoms but also by

[26] See E. Ackerknecht, *Malaria in the Upper Mississippi Valley,
1760–1900*, Baltimore, 1945, *passim*.

[27] C. E. Rosenberg, *The Cholera Years . . .* , Chicago, 1962, *passim*.

[28] Shryock, *The National Tuberculosis Association . . .* , New York,
1957, Chapter 2.

correlating these signs with lesions found at autopsy, much clearer entities could be discovered. Encouraged by surgeons who had always dealt with obvious injuries a new generation of physicians in post-Revolution Paris began to investigate such "structural pathology." To do this they had (1) to treat hundreds of patients, (2) improve the observation of symptoms, and (3) perform systematic autopsies. Encouraged by physical scientists to be objective, even in dealing with human subjects, these medical innovators—backed by the State—took over control of hospital services and made these institutions into centers of research.

Between 1800 and 1840 observation was improved by new instruments (such as the stethoscope), and by new methods (notably the use of clinical statistics). The older theorizing was repudiated as speculative, and vague "clinical pictures" were broken down into more specific entities—as when "inflammation of the chest" was resolved into bronchitis, pleurisy, pneumonia, and so on. Such findings, at the time, had little value for therapy; indeed, the critical approach tended to make scientists skeptical of old treatments and encouraged a "medical nihilism" which left healing largely to Nature. Advancing chemistry did, however, enable Paris pharmacists to isolate the active principles in vegetable drugs —as in producing quinine from cinchona during the 1820's— and so they were able to aid the practice of medicine in a limited manner. The work of "the Paris school" may be viewed as the advent of strictly modern medicine, for the hospitals of that city provided the first environment in which a present-day doctor would have felt in some degree at home.[29]

Developments in Paris and similar trends in London,

[29] Among the many works relating to the Paris school, see, e.g., M. Fosseyeaux, *Paris Médicale en 1830,* Paris, 1930, *passim,* and any good text covering modern medical history. Note also O. Temkin, "The Role of Surgery in the Rise of Modern Medical Thought," *Bull. Med. Hist.,* XXV, 1951, 248 ff.; and H. Guerlac, "Some Aspects of Science During the French Revolution," *Scientific Monthly,* LXXX, 1955, 93 ff.

Dublin, and Vienna, ushered in a new medical dispensation which attracted thousands of physicians from abroad. Among them were young American doctors who returned to Boston, New York, and Philadelphia, after 1830, urging clinical-pathological studies and a rejection of speculative "systems" and heroic practice. A few of these men did good research in the Gallic manner, as when Dr. William Gerhardt distinguished typhus from typhoid fever at the Philadelphia General Hospital in 1837; but many others—like Osler's "Alabama student"—found the American environment frustrating. "Practical," equalitarian people of the Jacksonian era had no interest in research which could identify but neither prevent nor cure illness; and most doctors, as well as patients, were disinclined to abandon remedies which were "tried and true."[30] There was even some suspicion, as in England, of French clinicians as materialists and skeptics.

Gradually, however, better education, the example of the physical sciences, and perhaps echoes of clinical skepticism made for a popular revolt against excessive bleeding and purging. By 1850 these practices were declining, and by the '70's were largely abandoned. At the same time most patients wanted not merely "watchful waiting" but positive help from their doctors. Into the resulting vacuum rushed medical sectarians, who maintained all-explaining "systems" impressive to laymen and promised cures by milder methods. Chief among them were the homeopaths, followers of the German physician Hahnemann, who proclaimed that "like cures like" (drugs causing certain symptoms would cure disease exhibiting these symptoms)—particularly, if given in minute doses in such pleasant forms as water or sugar pills.

Certain native sects also became popular, notably Thom-

---

[30] On the American reaction to the Paris school, see E. Ackerknecht, "Elisha Bartlett and the Philosophy of the Paris Clinical School," *Bull. Med. Hist.*, XXIV, 1950, 43 ff.; Shryock, *The Development of Modern Medicine*, New York, 1947, pp. 171–77.

sonianism which used mild, vegetable remedies. Meantime, health cults appeared which made a secular religion of hygiene, for which devotees were willing to endure such austere practices as vegetarianism or week-end bathing. Most physicians repudiated both sects and cults as "irregular" but found it impossible to suppress them. If Americans were entitled to religious freedom, why not medical freedom as well?

The invasion of medical practice by sectarians came at an unfortunate time for the "regulars." It encouraged the states to ignore or even repeal early licensing laws, so that medical schools of any sort could secure charters and authorize graduates to practice. And since education was cheap (involving only lectures and a few books), even "regulars" formed schools which admitted any literate student and made a "doctor" in less than a year. Although the "M.D." had originally been viewed with awe, this degree was so cheapened by 1850 that some medical leaders wanted to abandon it altogether.[31]

What were actually being produced were many second-rate medical men, who tended to serve the poorer or more isolated patients. Europeans also trained such personnel, but labeled them distinctly as apothecaries or *officiers de santé* and limited their activities. Democratic Americans, however, would allow no distinctions, addressed all practitioners as "doctor," and permitted them to engage in any sort of practice—as is largely true to this day.

Inadequate background and mediocre training were factors in the bad reputation of some medical students, who were

[31] W. F. Norwood, *Medical Education in the United States before the Civil War*, Phila., 1944, *passim;* see also the almost forgotten work by D. A. Gorton, *The History of Medicine . . .* , II, New York, 1904, Chapter 16; Shryock, "Public Relations of the Medical Profession . . . ," *Annals of Medical History*, new ser., II, 1930, 315–29; and "Sylvester Graham and the Popular Health Movement, 1830–1870," *Miss. Valley Hist. Rev.*, XVIII, 1931, 172–83.

condemned in newspapers as "crude, coarse, and ignorant." Moreover, by European standards, there were always too many practitioners and the resulting competition among them was keen. Even leading doctors engaged in abusive quarrels, especially in cases involving rivalries within faculties or competition between schools. An extreme example was that of the able but cantankerous Charles Caldwell of the Transylvania College. When he attacked a colleague for setting up a rival school at Louisville in 1834, the latter retorted that:

> We have stifled the barking of their curs, but now . . . we hear the . . . cry of their unkennelled bloodhound, who is to . . . achieve our destruction. But to speak less figuratively, Dr. Caldwell . . . has come out in a pamphlet . . . filled with abuse which in malice, hatred, virulence, and vindictiveness, has never been surpassed.[32]

Such exchanges did little for solidarity within the regular profession when it was most needed.

One by-product of this confusion, however, had its merits. The ease of getting charters for medical schools, many of which were proprietary, at least made possible by 1850 the first medical college for women. Gradually driven out of general practice after 1700, and even out of midwifery after 1800, women—encouraged by current feminism—began a long struggle to regain access to the medical field. By the '70's, however, European schools were beginning to accept "doctoring ladies" more readily than were the American.[33]

What with apparent decadence in their own schools and growing competition with sectarians, the status of the regular

[32] Quoted in W. F. Norwood, "American Education . . . to the Civil War," *Jour. Med. Education*, XXXII, June, 1957, 440. See also Caldwell's *Autobiography*, Phila., 1855, *passim*.
[33] Shryock, "Women in American Medicine," *Jour. of the Amer. Medical Women's Asso.*, V, Sept., 1950, 371–79; J. Steudel, "Heilkundige Frauen des Abendlandes," *Zentralblatt für Gynäkologie*, Heft 8, 1959, s. 284 ff.

medical profession seemed to be declining. In retrospect, however, this is open to question. True, there were many cheap schools and poorly-trained "doctors" during this era. But in 1800, in comparison, most practitioners had enjoyed no formal training whatever. By the '50's they still retained the old (though dubious) apprenticeships and had in addition at least a bowing acquaintance with formal education. Professional leaders were probably raising their sights and so forgot the even lower levels of earlier years. Although the American Medical Association, founded 1847, long failed in its immediate objective of reforming education, it at least provided a forum for critics and a potential pressure-group for the future.[34]

It may be added that, despite the difficulties mentioned, American medical men did make a few notable contributions to medical practice—especially in the field of surgery. Outstanding were technical improvements in dentistry and in gynecology, and the introduction of inhalation anesthesia (ether) by dentists in the 1840's—an innovation which was not only humane but of great aid to surgeons throughout the world.[35] Those who would ascribe these surgical contributions to native practicality or to "frontier individualism," however, should recall that surgery advanced only in the wake of progress in Britain and France, and often in the hands of men actually trained in those countries.

[34] See *American Medical Conventions, New York, 1846, Philadelphia, 1847,* Phila., 1847, *passim.* A few medical leaders of the '50's, instead of bemoaning "decline," hailed professional progress; e. g., W. Hooker, "The Present Mental Attitude and Tendencies of the Medical Profession," *New Englander,* X, 1852, 557 f. See also W. H. King, ed., *History of Homoeopathy . . . in America,* I, New York, 1905, 281.

[35] The discovery of anesthesia is an oft-told tale, but see especially V. Robinson, *Victory Over Pain . . . ,* New York, 1946; and the *Jour. of Med. Hist. . . . ,* I, Fall, 1946, primarily devoted to this theme. Most Europeans ignored, or took a dim view of, American medical achievements before 1890. But see, for recent historical appreciation, P. Diepgen, *Geschichte der Medizin . . . ,* II, Hälfte I, Berlin, 1949, 205.

In 1800 to 1850 Americans shared with Europeans the growing effort to deal with mental illness in a more scientific and humane manner. Rush had published the pioneer native work on psychiatry in 1812. He attempted therein to classify types of insanity, but ascribed all of them to "pervading vascular tension." Between 1820 and 1850 early asylums were founded, and their medical superintendents—our first psychiatrists—waxed optimistic over the cures achieved by "moral" treatments. Inspired by the same outlook, Dorothea Dix crusaded effectively for the founding of many state asylums. But psychiatrists, always confronted by the perplexing dichotomy of mind and body, had no such firm ground under foot as was provided in somatic medicine. Hence, they alternated between psychologic and somatic approaches, and by the 1870's tended to return to a physical orientation. Mental diseases were to be identified in the same manner as in general pathology. Meantime, many of the mentally ill—despite well-intentioned efforts—were concealed in homes, languished in jails, or "went over the hill" to the local poor house.[36]

The Civil War, much as it aroused the whole country, had little bearing on medicine. Sanitary conditions in camps were at first disgraceful, and deaths by disease—as in earlier wars—exceeded those in combat. Later, sanitation and hospital services were improved, especially in the more prosperous North; but—lacking aseptic knowledges—surgery was helpless in the presence of penetrating wounds. Even a large percentage of amputation cases were lost through infection. The chief scientific contribution of the war was the collection of data on the pathology of camp diseases and of major wounds, all of which was of little comfort at the time. This

---

[36] H. Deutsch, n. 21 above, Chapters 6–13; Helen Marshall, *Dorothea Dix . . .* , Chapel Hill, N.C., 1937, *passim;* N. Dain, *Concepts of Insanity in the United States, 1789–1865,* New Brunswick, N.J., 1964, Chapters 3–10.

war, indeed, occurred just too soon for doctors to take advantage of remarkable progress in German medicine which began in the 1850's but did not come to fruition until the '70's.[37]

⌐/

The advent of truly "modern medicine" is popularly ascribed to the half-century which followed 1870. One still hears the remark that "no one had thought of germs" before Pasteur. Actually, ideas which came to fruition in this era had been planted during earlier decades or even earlier centuries. Thus, the concept of pathogenic "germs" was well-known by the early 1700's—it was maintained by Cotton Mather—and was even somewhat "dated" by 1850. This theory had been revived from time to time, but could not be proved until better microscopes and laboratory techniques became available.[38] Equally essential was a clearer identification of disease entities, for causal factors could not be found for a disease not yet recognized. Even a Pasteur could never have found organisms responsible for so vague a condition as "inflammation of the chest."

Studies of parasitology and bacteriology, begun as early as the 1830's, had attracted increasing attention during the '40's and '50's, and assumed practical implications by the '60's. During the latter decade Pasteur's ideas about bacteria in fermentation were applied by Lister to the prevention of surgical infections. The latter did not have to know *what* organisms were responsible, he had only to use a carbolic acid spray ("antiseptic") to prevent *any* infection. The results

[37] Shryock, "A Medical Perspective on the Civil War," *Amer. Quarterly*, XIV, Summer, 1962, 161–73.

[38] On American contributions to such revivals, see John Crawford's essays in the *Observer and Repertory*, Baltimore, 1807; and Phyllis Allen (Richmond), "Etiological Theory in America Prior to the Civil War," *Jour. of the History of Med.* . . . , II, 1947, 489–520.

were most encouraging in that they removed the last major obstacle to surgery in general. By the 1880's, antiseptic and then aseptic methods were adopted in all advanced countries, and surgery moved from the periphery toward the center of medical practice.[39]

To discover the agents of specific diseases was more difficult, for here—as had long been surmised—one had to find the particular "germs" involved. But during the 1870's both Pasteur and Koch proved that the anthrax bacillus was an essential factor in the cause (etiology) of that disease. Employing the so-called "Koch's postulates," and his solid media for cultivating isolated species, French and German bacteriologists identified (1875–1900) the organisms involved in many of the most serious infections (cholera, typhoid, tuberculosis, and so on). Although few cures were found for another half-century, implications for preventive measures were soon apparent.[40]

A by-product of bacteriology, meantime, was the fact that identification of specific organisms provided a third and most helpful criterion for identification. Even if a patient displayed the symptoms *and* lesions usually observed in diphtheria, that disease was not present unless the causative bacteria were also found. This distinction was not merely academic; it might make all the difference in treatment as well as in prognosis.

During the preceding era, 1820–1870, emphasis had shifted from the doctrine of contagion to another old theory that infections were spread by "airs and waters"; hence, it followed that such diseases could be better controlled by sanitation than

[39] See J. D. Comrie, *History of Scottish Medicine*, II, Edinburgh, 1932, 635 ff.; D. Guthrie, *Lord Lister*, Baltimore, 1949, pp. 59 ff.

[40] Useful summaries of the emergence of bacteriology after 1870 are given in A. C. Abbott, *Principles of Bacteriology*, Phila., 1915, pp. 267 ff. (based on German sources); and in E. P. Gorham, "The History of Bacteriology," in M. P. Ravenel, ed., *A Half Century of Public Health*, New York, 1921, pp. 66–93.

by quarantines. Local health departments debated these two theories (1800 to 1850) but by the latter date British experience convinced Americans that "clean ups" of water supplies, streets, and sewage were the answer. Was not an ounce of prevention better than a pound of cure—especially when there was no cure? State health agencies supplemented the local departments of large cities after 1870. In 1872 The American Public Health Association was founded; and in 1879 Congress even created an able but short-lived National Board of Health.[41]

Sanitary reform had real value but was an empirical program. It was led chiefly by statisticians and engineers, and operated blindly as far as any given disease was concerned. But as soon as the typhoid bacillus was known and traced to water and food, doctors, co-operating with engineers, learned just how to protect the public against it. The same was true where insects were found to be vectors of such plagues as malaria and yellow fever. Meantime, in the case of tuberculosis, the denial of contagion had led doctors to ascribe it to heredity. But Koch's discovery of the tubercle bacillus revived the view that "T.B." was infectious after all. This opened up at least possibilities of prevention or cure.[42]

By about 1905, after the usual delays on all levels of government, control of water or food supplies and of insect vectors began to check typhoid, cholera, yellow fever, and malaria by preventing the organisms involved from reaching the public. In consequence death rates from these diseases dropped precipitately; for example, typhoid mortality in New

[41] G. Rosen, *A History of Public Health,* New York, 1958, Chapter 6; Shryock, "Origins . . . of the Public Health Movement in the United States," *Annals of Med. Hist.*, new ser., I, 1929, 645–65. Shryock, "Medicine and Society in the 19th Century," *Jour. of World Hist.* [UNESCO], V, 1959, 135–39.

[42] Shryock, *The National Tuberculosis Association . . . ,* Chapters 1–3.

York City fell from forty per 100,000 population in 1870 to about two in 1920.[43]

Tuberculosis mortality, strangely enough, began declining in England as early as 1850, and in "the States" after 1880, for no clearly known reason. In three large American cities, for example, this death rate was almost 400 per 100,000 in 1880, but dropped to 100 by 1920—before really effective measures had been taken against it. Here, again, a continuing rise in living standards was probably a factor. So much fear of the disease had finally been aroused, however, that local and state anti-tuberculosis societies were formed (1900–1925) and also a federated, National Tuberculosis Association in 1904.

These were voluntary bodies in which laymen and doctors co-operated in seeking means of prevention or cure for this one disease—a new type of health program which flourished most in America. Similar societies were eventually formed to combat cancer (1913), heart disease (1922), poliomyelitis (1938), and other diseases. These organizations did some valuable pioneer work, but by the 1940's they were criticized as over-specialized or competitive, and their roles have been taken over in some degree by official agencies.[44]

So much progress was made by 1920 against the diseases mentioned, that at long-last medical science began to have a real impact on public health. The best evidence of this is not only the declining mortality from specific diseases but also the acceleration in the rise of life expectancy at birth after 1900. Continued improvement in living conditions could not entirely account for this phenomenon.[45] In 1900 average life

[43] See e.g., the various papers in Ravenel, n. 40 above.

[44] Shryock, n. 42 above, pp. 269–75. A History of the National Foundation for Infantile Paralysis [now The National Foundation] has been prepared by S. Bennison, but not yet published,

[45] This was already realized in the 1920's; see, e.g., C.-E. A. Winslow, Chapter 8, in C. A. Beard, ed., *Whither Mankind,* New York, 1928—a critical study of death rates in New Haven, Conn., 1875–1925. Also,

expectancy had reached almost fifty years in the United States, having risen about ten years since 1850. But in the next half-century it rose to over sixty-eight years.[46]

As infectious diseases declined, however, the proportion of elderly survivors began to mount, and this was the most obvious reason for a rise in death rates from conditions associated with old age. Cancer mortality in New York City, for example, rose from 80 per 100,000 in 1920 to about 160 in 1940. Better reporting may have influenced these figures, but most authorities agreed that this disease was actually increasing.[47]

Difficulties were still encountered, moreover, in dealing with infections, as was demonstrated by the terrible influenza-pneumonia pandemic of 1917–18. Not until about 1910 was it realized that some infections were caused by ultra-microscopic organisms ("viruses" in the modern sense), and such entities were difficult to identify or to control. In certain cases, as in yellow fever, protection against vectors supplied a solution; but this was not possible with most respiratory diseases. In one case, however, a second line of defense had long been available; that is, vaccination against smallpox. It was at first easier to prepare vaccines against bacterial diseases; but eventually vaccines were discovered against other viral infections besides smallpox—such as "polio" and influenza.

It will be noted that defenses against infectious disease were now developing in depth. The first and most effective line was that which prevented an infection from reaching the public,

Winslow's, *The Conquest of Epidemic Diseases* . . . , Princeton, N.J., 1943, Chapters 11, 12, 17, and 18.

[46] *Historical Statistics of the United States, 1789–1945*, p. 45; and *Continuation to 1952 of Historical Statistics* . . . , p. 6, U.S. Bureau of the Census, Wash., D.C., 1949 and 1954.

[47] See, for early recognition of this trend, F. L. Hoffmann, *The Mortality from Cancer Throughout the World*, Newark, N.J., 1915, pp. 28 ff.

as in purifying water supplies. But if infection could not be avoided, men could be prepared in advance to resist effectively —either (1) by maintaining general good health, as through adequate nutrition, or (2) by means of either active immunizations (vaccination) or by passive immunization (use of activated serums "borrowed" from animals). A third line of defense, in case all else failed, was the one with which most doctors had always been concerned—the discovery of cures. A few new, specific drugs had been found during the nineteenth century—such as emetine against amoebic dysentery—but most therapy was simply ameliorative as late as 1910.

Fortunately, however, medical men had attained an increasingly reliable knowledge of structural pathology. They had proceeded from a study of gross organs to a study of tissues, and after 1860 to observation of the microscopic, constituent cells. Experimentation then began to reveal the reactions of cells to particular drugs, and so transcended the old trial-and-error approach to pharmacology. Systematic search could now be made for remedies against specific diseases, by scientists familiar with advancing biochemistry as well as pathology. The first positive result of such "rational" empiricism was Ehrlich's discovery of an arsenical called salvarsan ("606"), which proved (in 1910) to be a specific against syphilis. Although some twenty-five years were to elapse before other chemo-therapeutic agents were uncovered, the third line of defense was at least shown to be of promise for the future.[48]

Although the most obvious advances were made against infections, the era 1870–1920 also witnessed progress against deficiency diseases and even against certain degenerative entities as well. Experimental physiology and biochemistry

[48] See I. Galdston, *Behind the Sulfa Drugs,* New York, 1943, pp. 111 ff. For a concise bibliography covering medical developments 1820–1920, see sections by Gertrude L. Annan and Eileen R. Cunningham, in Janet Doe, ed., *A Handbook of Medical Library Practice,* Chicago, 1943, pp. 303 ff., 371 ff.

had reached a point by about 1900, at which deficiency conditions could be divided between those resulting from a lack of substances ingested by the body (malnutrition), and those caused by a failure of certain glands to produce so-called hormones *within* the body (endocrine disorders). In the case of malnutrition, old observations had shown that citrus juices would prevent scurvy; but a rational, biochemical approach (1880–1930) demonstrated the value of minute substances ("vitamins") in food which prevented such wide-spread, fatal diseases as beriberi and pellagra. The prevention and cure of the latter entity was as important for the southern states as was the increasing control of malaria.[49]

Progress in endocrinology, as in other fields, had its origin in the pathologic anatomy of 1800–1850; when lesions in endocrine glands were found to be associated with serious "clinical pictures." But as in nutritional studies, the resources of experimental physiology and biochemistry were needed to seek means of prevention or cure. By the 1890's experimental work on ductless glands led to the discovery that the thyroid produced a "thyroxine" so potent that the lack of only 3.5 grains per year made all the difference for the individual between complete imbecility and health. Moreover, if such a hormone were lacking, it could be supplied as a drug from animal sources. The most dramatic triumphs in this area were the discovery in 1922 of insulin as a treatment for diabetes (a disease resulting from failure of glands close to the pancreas); and the somewhat related discovery that the use of a liver diet could control the fatal "pernicious anemia." [50]

American scientists, chiefly members of medical faculties, played an important role in these advances after about 1885.

[49] See, e.g., R. G. Hoskins, "The Internal Secretions," in J. O. Stieglitz, *Chemistry in Medicine,* New York, 1928.

[50] See L. G. Stevenson's *Sir Frederick Banting,* Toronto, 1946; and G. W. Corner's *George Hoyt Whipple,* Phila., 1963, especially pp. 177–89.

One recalls for example, the research of Theobald Smith on the role of a secondary host in spreading infections (1889); of E. V. McCollum on vitamins A and B (1915); of J. J. Abel's isolation of the amazingly potent adrenalin (1898); and the cumulative studies of G. H. Whipple, C. S. Minot, and W. P. Murphy which led to the cure of pernicious anemia (1926). One also recalls the emerging leadership of American surgeons (after 1890) as in the work of the brothers Mayo in Rochester, Minnesota; of W. S. Halstead in Baltimore; and of Harvey Cushing in Boston and New Haven. The Mayos advanced surgical diagnosis and techniques along many lines; Halstead related surgery closely to biologic research and checked the rather reckless practice which asepsis had made possible; and Cushing demonstrated the possibility of extending the province of surgery from the abdomen to the brain and other neurologic areas.

The first generation of American physicians who made their schools research centers—beginning with Johns Hopkins in 1893—were largely trained on the post-graduate level in German-speaking universities. Between 1870 and 1914 some 15,000 American doctors made this pilgrimage—surpassing the earlier migrations to Edinburgh, London, and Paris, even in proportion to population.

Advancing science made specialization in practice inevitable, and most of the Americans who flocked to Vienna, Munich, and Berlin sought quick training in a specialty; but a few worked for years at Strasbourg, Zurich, or Breslau in basic research. In the German cities they observed full-time professorships, fine facilities in hospitals and "labs," *Lehrfreiheit* and *Lehrnfreheit,* and a general enthusiasm for original investigations.[51] Returning to "the States," they thought prospects in both education and research as dim as had their grandfathers

[51] T. N. Bonner, *American Doctors and German Universities,* Lincoln, Nebraska, 1963, Chapters 2–4.

returning from Paris fifty years before. But two circumstances made the situation after 1885 quite different.

In the first place, medical science now offered means for preventing and even a hope for curing disease, instead of the nihilism of earlier decades. Here was a promise which the most practical person could appreciate. In the second place, rapid industrial development led to mounting wealth, and certain millionaires decided to contribute generously to the support of a promising medical science—just when the costs of good hospitals and schools were necessarily rising.

German-trained leaders in the better medical schools (Hopkins, Harvard, Michigan) found the continued mediocrity of medical education intolerable. Medical professors in this country still retained private practice, although incomes from apprentices vanished when this practice declined, after 1870, with the lengthening of the curriculum. Hence, professors were able to infiltrate the medical societies as practitioners, and appealed to the A.M.A. (American Medical Association) to reform the schools. The latter, because of their power to license, were primarily responsible for the low state of both training and practice; and the reformers—consciously or unconsciously—returned to an earlier program in appealing for control by medical societies. The latter, in turn, succeeding in persuading most states to re-establish the examining and licensing boards which had earlier been abandoned; and such bodies (1875 to 1900) were able to exert some pressure for better educational standards. By 1900, moreover, liberals in the A.M.A. secured its reorganization, and in 1904 set up a Council on Education which began to rate the various schools.

Unfortunately, the many A.M.A. members who represented poor schools still constituted a built-in opposition to reform, and it was difficult in any case to secure either the funds or co-operation needed for systematic rating programs.

Moreover, there was still some popular suspicion of "regulars" who were critical of sectarian or even of proprietary colleges. At this point, fortunately, one of the major foundations set up by philanthropists after 1900—the Carnegie Foundation for the Advancement of Teaching—employed the able, and critical, Abraham Flexner to survey all medical schools. His devastating *Report* of 1910, prepared by a layman for a lay body, could not be blamed on any professional desire for a "monopoly," and the response of both the public and the universities was prompt and effective.

Between 1910 and '20 weak schools (including most of the sectarian and also of the non-university schools) closed, or were merged, all over the country. This final victory for the A.M.A., after sixty years of intermittent efforts, was related in both cause and effect to general advances in education, to German influences and research, and to rising standards in practice. One consequence of this upheaval was that the few sectarian schools which survived, did so because homeopathy was reabsorbed into regular medicine—a process which a later sect, osteopathy, now also seems to be following.[52]

In raising the standards of medical education the A.M.A. co-operated with a National Confederation of State Medical Examining Boards (1891), and with a Confederation of Reciprocity (1902) which sought to persuade state boards to accept out-of-state licenses. In 1912 these two bodies merged to form the present Federation of State Medical Boards. Meantime, the Association of American Medical Colleges (1890) became the chief representative of the schools as such, but made no effort to recapture licensing powers for these institutions. Indeed, all these organizations were co-operating,

[52] Flexner alone should not be credited with the reorganizations following 1910; he provided the final push which enabled the A.M.A. to get over the hump blocking reform. More than any one man, however, he precipitated the ensuing developments; see his *I Remember*, New York, 1940, *passim*.

by 1920, in the A.M.A. Council's continuing program for rating the schools through regular inspections. The great improvement in medical education (1910–1925) gradually led to a parallel rise in standards of practice; so that "the safe general practitioner" at last began to emerge.[53]

This era was the great turning point in the history of American medicine. After three centuries of colonial dependence on European science, American research attained a status equal to that of the better European centers. After an equally long period of mediocre or inferior training, medical education also attained a level similar to that reached in the Old World. And last but not least, the average practice of the younger, native physicians became at least as reliable as that of their counterparts in western Europe.

These developments, nevertheless, should not be viewed in a chauvinistic or otherwise complacent manner. It is, first of all, a chastening thought that similar, basic "medical reform" had been achieved in German-speaking countries by the 1850's, and in the United Kingdom by 1900, or 1910. Second-class doctors, so-labeled, largely disappeared in Germany by the 1870's, in France by the 1890's, and in the United Kingdom by 1920; but were still around in "the States"—indistinguishable by title—as late as the 1930's.

One might even reverse the attitude usually taken toward "the Flexner era," by replacing praise with the question: Why did these reforms not occur earlier? (In historical studies, the common question as to why things happened when they did, is often no more significant than the query: Why not at some earlier point in time?) In this case, as usual, there is no simple answer, but certain partial explanations are obvious.

---

[53] Summarized accounts of these developments will be found in D. F. Smiley, "History of the Association of American Medical Colleges," *Jour. Med. Ed.*, vol. 32, 1957, pp. 512–18; W. L. Bierring, "Medical Licensure After Forty Years," *Conn. State Med. Jour.*, vol. 20, 1956, pp. 724–29.

The vast size of the United States by 1850, its regional divisions leading to Civil War, its heterogeneous population, and the complexity of its federal type of government, all may have delayed professional progress. Problems must have been simpler, in some respects, in such smaller and more homogeneous countries as Denmark and Holland, or even in France and the United Kingdom. Traditional dependence on Europe in science as well as in other matters—a heritage of colonial days —was also not easy to overcome.

Indifference to research also may be ascribed to the practicality of a people absorbed in "conquering a continent," to whom technology naturally seemed more significant than "pure" science.[54] In some degree, a similar attitude obtained in Britain, which was likewise involved in developing large new areas—in this case, as it happened, overseas. Americans inherited from the mother country, moreover, the "voluntary" tradition in professional and educational matters which, though not without merit, made difficult any prompt, systematic reform.

Last but not least, as Tocqueville had pointed out long before, equalitarianism after 1830 denied to Americans the aristocratic patrons or governments which at times supported basic science in Europe. It was not until after 1900 that some of these factors were overcome or, as in the case of a more useful, applied medicine, simply disappeared in America as a result of trans-Atlantic progress.

One may also qualify the optimism of 1920 by recalling that similar enthusiasm in 1820 was soon followed by disillusionment. Reactions after 1920 were not so extreme, particularly as advances in some fields were even more marked during subsequent decades. Yet still pertinent was the truism that in

[54] Shryock, "American Indifference to Basic Science During the Nineteenth Century," *Archives Internationales d'Histoire des Sciences,* no. 5, 1948, pp. 50–65.

solving some problems men often create others. If infectious diseases were controlled, the degenerative diseases increased; if medical societies reformed the schools, the latter in turn soon found themselves fettered by the very requirements which had once set them free. And a restored, public confidence in medicine was achieved only by more expensive education, specialization, and equipment which necessarily raised medical costs. Thus, in solving one difficulty in public relations— distrust of practice—the profession substituted the equally troublesome problems of "medical care." All of this, however, relates more to the era after 1920 than to that which preceded it.

The recent decades will be treated here briefly for several reasons; to wit: the sources become overwhelming, perspectives on things contemporary are foreshortened, and, finally, many a reader will be more familiar with the intricacies of given developments than can be any single author. Nevertheless, certain major trends and current problems may be mentioned in conclusion.

After 1920 research continued central to all medical progress, not only in pathology and therapeutics but also in the whole social mechanism that promoted the understanding, prevention, or cure of illness. It was the stone thrown into the social pond, which in turn produced ripples in ever-widening circles. But, to continue this figure, one must recall what motives led to the throwing of the stone, and under what circumstances? These latter questions led to studies in the psychology and sociology of research, in medicine as in other fields, and made the whole process more self-conscious than ever before.

Investigations accelerated, as progress encouraged large foundations to give increasing funds to medical scientists—

first in terms of "block grants" which endowed institutes or schools, later in the form of time-limited aid to individuals. The Rockefeller Foundation alone, between 1910 and 1940, extended to medicine and public health, funds totaling almost $170 million—the greater part of it to American institutions. In so doing, the several Rockefeller boards often pioneered in certain areas, as in founding at Hopkins in 1916 the first School of Hygiene, and in supporting at the same university in 1913 the first full-time clinical professorships.[55] By 1940 medicine and public health became the greatest beneficiaries of private foundations: in that year it was estimated that this field received about $9.5 million, in comparison with some $3.7 million allocated to all other "natural sciences." [56] Yet as late as 1896 the total endowment of all native medical schools had not exceeded some $500,000. Medicine thus provides the best illustration of the "Cinderella" role in the history of American science.

Funds from foundations began to decline shortly before 1940, however, though this was not the chief explanation of the great shift after 1945 to federal support. In both of these connections financial aid was not an unmixed blessing, because a fear grew that bodies outside the universities might—directly or indirectly—control the direction in which research moved. On the whole, however, both foundation and federal aid were essential to the advance of medical science. Sometimes the academic men who directed these agencies could anticipate needs sooner than could conservative universities; and even though the former doubtless made mistakes, in the long run such "outside" aid was a major factor in the growing

[55] S. and J. T. Flexner, *William Henry Welch* . . . , New York, 1941, pp. 266 f.; Shryock, *The Unique Influence of the Johns Hopkins University on American Medicine,* Copenhagen, 1953, pp. 38–42, 47–53; A. Flexner, *I Remember,* pp. 176 ff.

[56] Geneva Seybold, *American Foundations and their Fields,* New York, 1942, pp. 38 f.

prestige of native medical science in the years 1930–1960. Prior to the first of these years no native American had won a Nobel prize in medical fields, but thereafter they led all the rest.

Actual motivations in research, in medicine as in other areas, varied widely. Commercial firms, including the drug houses which spent large sums on applied medicine, naturally were concerned with profits. "Pure" scientists were influenced by current social needs (the dangers, or drama, of a particular disease), promising leads already open in certain areas, funds available, publicity, and so on. There was even some waste, bluff, or inefficiency as research facilities proliferated, but the proportion of this sort of thing never bulked very large.[57] The chief difficulty caused by accelerated studies was the rapid expansion of knowledge, which made a doctor's practice, learned in one decade, out of date by the next. Efforts to help "obsolete" practitioners through "refresher" programs in schools or hospitals have been only partially successful.

In the basic medical discipline, pathology, interest was transferred from structural to functional problems—from the discovery of cells to a study of how cells *behaved*. Structure, however, was never overlooked; and was indeed revived in a sense by one of the most remarkable of all the instruments of observation used in medicine—the electron microscope of the '40's. Thereafter, the investigation of structure reached down not only into cells as such, but into cell constituents and even into molecular phenomena.

The physical sciences, gradually realizing the dreams of the 1600's, also contributed other instruments useful to pathologists, as when the photography of the 1840's was followed by the moving pictures of the 1920's. The contributions of

[57] The classic indictment of this aspect of the story is the Sinclair Lewis–Paul de Kruif novel, *Arrowsmith*, New York, 1931, though all of it is not to be taken at face value.

biochemistry to physiology have already been mentioned; and these were followed by such equally valuable aids from biophysics as the invention of the electrocardiograph, the electroencephalograph, and the whole study of the physical-chemical nature of nerve impulses.

Another interesting trend in pathology was a revived interest in the old concept of generalized disease states and body functions. The phenomena of immunology, of endocrinology, of genetics, and of psychosomatic relationships all indicated that disease was rarely entirely localized or completely specific in nature. The concept of specificity continued to be essential for public health and to some extent in therapy; but terms considered old fashioned in 1900 (such as "constitutional factors," "hereditary predispositions," or "psychosomatic relations") once more invaded the literature.

In the meantime, psychiatrists were rewarded by the discovery of a somatic basis for certain mental disorders, notably the syphilis of paresis and the arteriosclerosis of "senile dementia." On the whole, however, they were disillusioned by the anatomic research ("brain mythology") carried over from physical medicine (1850–1900). This reaction, in turn, encouraged a revival of psychological approaches which attained its most extreme and popular form in the psychoanalysis of Sigmund Freud. Signs are already appearing in the '60's, however, that there is again disillusionment in this area. Whether the literary men and social scientists, who likewise welcomed "analysis" as an *avant garde* revelation, will also regain some balance is still open to question.[58] Meantime, the

[58] Shryock, *Development of Modern Medicine*, New York, 1947, Chapter 17. Cf. S. Freud, *A General Introduction to Psychoanalysis*, transl. by G. S. Hall, New York, 1920; C. Landis "Psychoanalysis and Scientific Method," Amer. Philosophical Soc. *Proceeds.*, vol. 84, 1941, pp. 515 ff.; and such recent comments as those of Dr. S. S. Kety, in the *Proceeds.*, Sixth Annual Conference on Graduate Medical Education, Univ. of Penna., Phila., 1964, pp. 41, 44.

renewal of somatic studies, on an empirical level, led to the discovery of drugs of some promise in psychiatric treatment.

Therapy in general took "a great leap forward" when long-continued efforts to emulate Ehrlich led to the development of the sulpha drugs in the late 1930's and of the antibiotics early in the next decade. Both types of materials had been known earlier, but were not finally demonstrated and produced in quantity until the years noted. The origins of these drugs are to be credited to German, British, and French investigators, although American pharmaceutical firms made the first effective antibiotic (penicillin) available during World War II.

Sulpha drugs and antibiotics revealed remarkable curative properties, and for a range of diseases which otherwise had little in common. Thus, the "sulphas" were more or less effective against pneumonia, meningitis, erysipelas, mastoid infections, gonorrhea, and so on. The antibiotics were similarly versatile, and it is not strange that men spoke of a major "break through" and of "wonder-drugs." Many of these materials proved to be bacteriostatic rather than strictly bacteriocidal ("magic bullets") but were none the less effective for that reason. Their use not only greatly lowered mortality from many infections, but made unnecessary earlier forms of therapy which were more complex or dangerous. Resort to serums declined, for example, and mastoid operations all but disappeared.[59]

As in the case of earlier substances once hailed as cure-alls (from tobacco to quinine), limitations and dangers did subsequently appear. Certain of the drugs, in unusual cases, had dangerous "side effects" in terms of little-understood, allergic reactions. The use of penicillin, indeed, occasionally proved fatal. Moreover, various bacteria developed immunities against the commonly used antibiotics—perhaps through a rapid

[59] Shryock, *American Medical Research* . . . , Chapter 4.

evolution involving a "survival of the fittest." At times, research seemed to involve a race between these mutating organisms and men who were seeking to keep one jump ahead of them with new "biologicals." Outstanding, in the latter connection, was S. Waksman's discovery of streptomycin—so effective against the long-resistant tubercle bacillus—but even this drug has had to be used in combination with potent chemotherapy.[60]

Biochemistry produced other potent and versatile drugs by the 1930's. Work on the cortex of the adrenal glands, for example, led E. C. Kendall to isolate the hormone cortin in crystalline form, and various steroids were subsequently secured from the same source. In 1949 Kendall, P. S. Hench, and others showed that one of these, cortisone, was remarkably useful in treating serious forms of arthritis. A related hormone (A.C.T.H.) has also been used in combination with cortisone against various diseases;[61] and these products at times exhibited the curious effect of suppressing symptoms (to the patient's relief) without "curing" the underlying pathology. Here again, however, precautions had to be taken against side effects.

It is impossible to outline all the advances in chemotherapy in this era, some of which—such as new drugs found for controlling high blood pressure, or for preventing clotting after surgery or coronary occlusion—were of great value. But, in general, one may say that this era witnessed a return to a dependence on medication after nearly a century of skepti-

---

[60] Shryock, *The National Tuberculosis Association* . . . . , pp. 252–54, 298–300. See, as more essential, Dr. Waksman's own publications on these developments.

[61] C. Singer and E. A. Underwood, *A Short History of Medicine*, 2 ed., New York and Oxford, 1962, pp. 540, 548. A critical survey of American research in the 1950's is provided in Esther E. Lape, ed., *Medical Research; A Midcentury Survey*, 2 vols. (Amer. Foundation), Boston, 1955, *passim*.

cism.[62] A similar dependence on advancing surgery was also apparent. The major trends here were the further development of neurologic, as well as of abdominal, operations and, by the '30's, the surgical invasion of the thoracic area. Technology was especially vital in this latter step in that much depended on the invention of such devices as artificial heart and kidney machines. Currently, there is much interest in the actual replacement of heart valves and arteries, and in the possible transplantation of entire organs.

The outward and visible sign of confidence in drugs was the growth of the pharmaceutical industry, which reflected much more than the general trend toward "big business." By the 1920's the "ethical" firms were larger and more influential than the so-called patent-medicine (proprietary) companies; since the latter—along with individual quacks—were gradually inhibited by A.M.A.-inspired federal "food and drug" legislation.

The first real federal law in this field, promoted by the late Harvey Wiley, was passed in 1906; and this was tightened up against the dangers of potent new drugs in 1938. Further acts were passed in 1952 and 1962. Indeed, it is now thought by some pharmacologists that regulations are actually too strict, in that it may cost as much as $150,000 today to meet requirements for placing a new drug on the market.[63]

The regulation of food and drugs was but one aspect of the continuing expansion of federal activities in the health field. The origins of such interest can be traced back to about 1800,

[62] See, e.g., the enlightening papers by Waksman, Temkin, Stevenson, Rappleye, and others, in, I. Galdston, *The Impact of the Antibiotics on Medicine and Society*, N.Y. Academy of Medicine, 1958, *passim*. On the history of both pharmaceutical education (an important story in itself) and industry, see Kremer's and Urdang's *History of Pharmacy*, revised by G. Sonnedecker, 3 ed., Phila., 1963, Chapters 13–16.

[63] *Ibid.*, pp. 199–201; George Koelle, "Diseases Related to Chemical Agents . . . ," *Report of Proceeds.*, Sixth Annual Conference on Graduate Medical Education, Phila. (Univ. of Penna.), Dec., 1964, p. 64.

when the government had provided compulsory health insurance for merchant seamen in connection with the early marine hospitals. These institutions set up a laboratory in New York City in 1888 and moved it to Washington in 1891. In 1902 a research division was established, reports were issued, and it became apparent that a hospital system was being transformed into a health service. All this was recognized in 1908 by the adoption of the title "United States Public Health Service." The subsequent achievements of this Service cannot be followed here. But it should be noted that the National Institutes of Health began to be set up in Bethesda, Maryland, in 1930; and that, since World War II, congressional funds have enabled these centers to become the chief source of medical research funds for the entire country. Various other federal agencies, such as the Department of Agriculture and the military services, are also involved in medical investigations.[64] Not the least among these activities has been the evolution of the old U.S.A. Surgeon General's Library into the present National Medical Library, which is probably the greatest such institution in the world.

It is hardly necessary to add, in conclusion, that an era which witnessed such advances in medical research and practice also was characterized by striking changes and new problems relating to the medical profession. One of these has already been mentioned; that is, the conclusion reached by some as early as the 1930's that medical schools were now over-regulated by A.M.A. ratings and the requirements of state licensing boards. Recently, some faculties have even voiced a hope that licensing power could be returned once more to the schools, in order to permit free experimentation with curricula and educational methods.

[64] Shryock, *American Medical Research* . . . , pp. 268–73; A. Hunter Dupree, *Science in the Federal Government: A History of Policies and Activities to 1940*, Cambridge, Mass., 1957, *passim*.

This demand, however, has not become widespread, perhaps because of memories of the chaos of the days when schools *did* control licensing. It is also true that one of the chief difficulties in this area—the existence of fifty different, state examining boards—has been partly met by reciprocity agreements among them. Even more promising has been the development of the voluntary National Board of Medical Examiners, founded in 1915, whose carefully developed tests are now accepted in nearly all of the states.[65]

Certain problems persist, of course, such as the fact that real specialists—trained in hospital residencies—have no more legal authorization for working in their respective fields than does any general practitioner. The chief scandal here is the performance of the greater part of general surgery by general practitioners, who have not been certified by the voluntary, specialty boards which began to appear as early as 1916. Neither the state agencies nor the National Board have been inclined to take over any formal licensing of specialists.

Even more complex is the fact that when the number of medical schools was reduced (1910–1920), with a consequent decline in the number of graduates, the national population was expanding rapidly. The outcome by the 1930's was a decline in the proportion of doctors to population, which became extreme—by American standards—in the 1950's. The same thing was true of the supply of registered ("trained") nurses; and the consequent growth of ancillary personnel—technicians, therapists, practical nurses—has not fully filled the gap. When "medicare" goes into operation in 1966 this gap will yawn even wider.[66]

It is true that the proportion of doctors is still larger in the

[65] See N. A. Womack, "The Evolution of the National Board of Medical Examiners," unpub. article, n.d. (*ca.* 1960), Chapel Hill, N.C., pp. 12–15; Bierring, n. 53 above, *passim*.

[66] See, e.g., Howard Rusk, "Doctor Shortage Grows," *N.Y. Times*, Oct. 14, 1962.

United States than in even advanced countries in Europe—Sweden, and the United Kingdom—and that the latter show a slightly higher life expectancy at birth than does the American population. But traditional ratios between the numbers of doctors and patients cannot be changed too quickly without serious difficulties. In this context the United States has gone from an excess of practitioners in 1900 to a deficit in the 1960's.

Plans are now under way, therefore, to found a dozen or more new medical schools over the next decade, but this is necessarily a slow and costly procedure. Voices are once again raised in favor of reintroducing partially trained practitioners to take over the burden of routine work. As a last resort, this may become necessary; but—except in the case of midwives, long neglected in this country—such a step would present difficulties. Many adjustments would have to be made by schools and licensing bodies, and the whole program suggests a return to the long-discredited, second-grade "doctors" of earlier periods. What the public reaction would be is still unknown.

Schools and licensing boards, of course, are not the only institutions which have played major roles in promoting better training and practice over the past seventy-five years. Outstanding has been the gradual improvement of hospital administration and facilities, developed under the oversight of the American Hospital Association founded in 1898. Both this association and the national surgical societies did much to assure minimal standards in the once sadly mismanaged American hospitals. Co-operation to this end, between the hospital association and the American College of Surgeons, was inaugurated in 1916.[67] Surgeons in particular (after 1870) had to look to hospitals for training and practice; but all

[67] See, e.g., L. Davis, *Fellowship of Surgeons* . . . , Springfield, Ill., 1960, pp. 173–85.

medical students and nurses were likewise dependent on hospital-centered education. Residents, who were to become specialists, were located only in "teaching hospitals"; but many young graduates had to spend a year or more in independent hospitals as interns. Supposedly, this provided a fifth year of medical education, but often these beginners were given little supervision and so were exploited for their temporary services.

Even so, it became difficult to find enough graduates to fill all the vacancies, and in large cities many of these vacancies were taken over by interns of foreign (usually non-European) origin. This influx of foreign physicians, of unknown qualifications, confronted licensing authorities with special difficulties. Although some of these men came for advanced training —reversing the long history of American pilgrimages to European medical schools—others hoped to establish themselves in this country. Like native colleagues, few wished to enter general practice; but "group practice" may offer greater opportunities in the future.

Most pressing, among the public relations of the medical profession (1925–1965), was the problem of "medical care." Compulsory health insurance for the poor had been introduced in Germany by the 1880's and in the United Kingdom in 1911. At the latter time it was also seriously considered in this country—even by the A.M.A. and by state legislatures. But after World War I the A.M.A. established a policy of opposition maintained ever since that time. Without going into the arguments, pro and con, it may be said that by 1950 the United States was almost the only advanced country which lacked such a system. The depression of the 1930's revived a demand for insurance, but ensuing prosperity tended to discourage it. Despite President Truman's support, the program was defeated in the late 1940's, became dormant in the '50's, but was revived again in the '60's. The introduction of "medicare" for the elderly, in 1966, is widely viewed as a first step toward a general adoption of compulsory insurance as a special phase of broadening federal welfare activities. At present the A.M.A. seems inclined to co-operate, but there have been threats of a "doctors' strike," even as there were at times in both Germany and Britain.

Certain critics of American medicine declared, during the 1930's, that the nation led the world in scientific standards but lagged far behind in providing superior medical care to the mass of the people. However valid at the time, both of these comments would now appear exaggerated. Scientific standards in native education and practice are certainly among the highest in the world but are not always uniquely superior. And although some Americans still lack adequate care, this is often the result of shortages of personnel. Better procedures, meantime, are called for in adapting hospitals more intelligently to the psychology, as well as the technical needs, of patients. This is one of the points at which behavioral scientists can be of greatest aid in the medical environment.[68]

The greatest difficulty of recent decades, as noted, was caused by the rising costs of more complex, technical care, and the inability of many to pay for such care. This need is now beginning to be met, not only by "medicare" but also by the Veterans Bureau and by new federal welfare programs. Much remains to be done, in "medical care" as well as in scientific achievements; yet medicine—despite all its limitations, technical and professional—constitutes one of the few fields in which a good case still can be made for the nineteenth-century concept of progress.

[68] See, e.g., Esther L. Brown, *Newer Dimensions of Patient Care*, Pt. I, 1961, Pt. II, 1962, New York, *passim;* and, for the role of social scientists, other publications of the Russell Sage Foundation; and J. A. Clausen and R. Straus, eds., *The Annals* of the Amer. Acad. of Polit. and Soc. Science, vol. 346, March, 1963, papers on "Medicine and Society." On the advantages of "group" over "solo" practice, see *Medicine and the Changing Order*, New York (N.Y. Acad. of Med.), 1947, pp. 52 f., 137–41, 200 f., *passim.*

PERIOD PIECES

II

Medical Practice
in the Old South *

I

The Old South failed to keep step in progress, economically or culturally, with the Old North. Northerners blamed this on the South, in terms of climate and slavery; Southerners blamed it on the Yankees, in terms of tariff and abolitionism. Both theses were partly true, but both were exaggerated and incomplete. Other factors than those noted made for cultural lag in Dixie.

One of these was the disease situation, which varied somewhat in the two sections, and on the whole tended to be more serious in the South. Frontier conditions prevailed there to a greater degree, and such conditions were always conducive to malarial fevers, since there was little opportunity in new clearings to drain the land, or to determine the most healthful locations prior to settlement.[1] The longer summers

* Reprinted from *The South Atlantic Quarterly*, XXIX, No. 2, April, 1930—by permission.

[1] A detailed discussion of the conditions conducive to the "autumnal fevers" is given in Daniel Drake, *Principal Diseases of the Interior Valley of North America,* etc. (Cincinnati, 1850), pp. 709 ff., 819. There was a general tendency, as malaria decreased with the development of a settlement, for typhoid to take its place; but the two commonly overlapped. See, e.g., S. C. Farrar, "General Report on the . . . Diseases of Jackson, Miss.," in E. D. Fenner, (ed.) *Southern Medical Reports,* I. 349, 350, 357 (New Orleans, 1850).

and more steady heat of the South encouraged insect life associated with malaria, yellow fever, dengue, and typhoid; made more difficult the preservation of food; complicated sanitary problems; and was responsible for such a folk habit as going barefooted, which in turn resulted in hook-worm infection. Finally, the institution of slavery involved in some areas a routine diet which caused common parasitic infections, and—it may be—serious malnutrition diseases not yet definitely identified. Along the lower Mississippi and the Gulf, e.g., there obtained the dreaded *cachexia africana* or dirt-eating disease of the West Indies; which doubtless involved a severe form of hook-worm infection, but which in the writer's opinion was also suggestive at times of beri-beri.[2]

It is hardly necessary to elaborate upon the economic handicap suffered by the South as a result of these conditions.[3] A few Southern physicians had already begun, as early as 1850, to adopt the now common procedure of calculating losses by illness in terms of dollars and cents. It was claimed at that time, for example, that the cost of disease and death in New Orleans alone totaled about $45,000,000 annually, an average expense of $105 per capita. The mortality rate of this

[2] See, e.g., John Hunter, *Observations on the Diseases of the Army in Jamaica*, etc. (Lon., 3 ed., 1808), pp. 248–250; J. B. Dazille, *Observations sur les Maladies des Nègres*, etc. (Paris, 1776), I. 342 ff.; W. M. Carpenter, "Observations on the Cachexia Africana," etc., *New Orleans Med. Jour.*, I. 146–168 (1844); T. W. Craigin, "Observations on Cachexia Africana or Dirt-Eating," *Amer. Jour. of the Med. Sciences*, XXXIV, 356 ff. (1854); J. B. Duncan, "On the Diseases of the Parish of St. Mary, La.," *So. Med. Rep'ts.*, I. 194, 195; H. T. Catterall, *Judicial Cases Concerning American Negro Slavery* (Wash., 1926), I. 315, 342, 464. Cf. C. W. Stiles, *Report upon . . . Hookworm Disease in the United States* (Treasury Dept. Hygiene Laboratory Bull. No. 10, Wash., 1903), p. 36; and Edward B. Vedder, "Some Further Remarks on Beri-Beri," *Amer. Jour. of Tropical Diseases and Preventive Med.*, I. 826–847 (1914).

[3] The effect of hook-worm disease on the "poor whites" of the Old South, is noted in various works; see references in R. H. Shryock, *Georgia and the Union* (Durham, 1926), p. 75, n. 33.

city was estimated to be as high as 8.1 per cent of the population, which was almost three times the contemporary rates in London, New York, and Philadelphia.[4]

New Orleans, popularly known as "the graveyard of the Southwest," was of course a peculiarly horrible example. There were, in contrast, certain areas in the South such as the upper piedmont of the Carolinas and Georgia, or certain cities such as Charleston, in which the public health was reported to be quite "salubrious."[5] This may be accounted for by certain conditions which in part compensated the South for the disadvantages noted. The winters were obviously kind to the aged and the poor. Since there were few large cities, there were few slums and, presumably for this reason, one heard relatively little of typhus and the venereal diseases. The latter, however, were apparently common in towns of any size, and occasionally spread from them to the plantations.[6] Again, the upper piedmont and mountain areas were sufficiently high and dry to avoid most of the endemic fevers. Last, but not least, the South escaped some of the chronic drunkenness

[4] J. C. Simonds, "On the Sanitary Condition of New Orleans, Illustrated by Its Mortuary Statistics," *So. Med. Rep'ts.*, II (1851) 215, 231–237. It is of incidental interest that Simonds used slave values in calculating the value of whites lost by disease. *Cf.* Irving Fisher, *Report on National Vitality* (Wash., 1909), pp. 117 ff.

[5] J. G. de Roulhac Hamilton (ed.), *The Ruffin Papers*, IV. 133 (Raleigh, 1920); *So. Med. Rep'ts.*, II. 419; *Trans. Amer. Med. Asso.*, IX, 431–481 (1856); *Boston Med. and Surg. Jour.*, IV. 103 (1831); Josiah Nott, "Health and Longevity in the Southern Seaports," *Southern Jour. of Med. and Pharmacy*, II. 1 ff. (1847). Nott's article presents the best case for the relative salubrity of the South. See also J. D. B. De Bow, *Industrial Resources of the Southern and Western States*, II, 83–92.

[6] *So. Med. Rep'ts.*, I. 24; *So. Med. and Surg. Jour.*, III. 209 (1838), N. S., I. 16, 17, 682, 683 (1845); H. I. Catterall, *Judicial Cases Concerning American Negro Slavery*, II (Wash., 1929), 320, 321, 577. U. B. Phillips, *Life and Labor in the Old South*, (Boston, 1929), p. 321. *Cf. Practical Rules for the Management and Medical Treatment of Negro Slaves in the Sugar Colonies, By a Professional Planter* (Lon., 1811), pp. 348–353. Typhus also occurred at times in slave quarters; see J. D. B. De Bow, *Industrial Resources of the Southern and Western States*, New Orleans, 1852, II. 338.

which so complicated the disease problem of the Northern slum, in so far as masters displayed a vested interest in the sobriety of slaves.[7]

Statistical comparisons of the health of the sections were attempted as early as the 'forties, and while obviously unreliable, are interesting as expressions of a state of mind. One enterpising Northern authority[8] found, on the basis of the census of 1840, that of 100 babies born there would be alive at the end of five years:

In New Hampshire 94
In Massachusetts 85
In North Carolina 79.7
In Mississippi 72.5

These, or similar data, must have impressed the actuaries of the period, for life insurance companies were in the habit of charging one per cent more premium on Southern risks. Outsiders were certainly convinced that the South was a relatively dangerous country. Of course they exaggerated, as in the case of the observer who solemnly declared in 1795 that no native of "Petersborough [Virginia] had ever lived beyond the age of twenty-one years."[9] Yet the Southern people themselves had their misgivings and were prone to view the North as a promised land of health, to which those of means escaped each year during the summer season.

In view of all these circumstances, it is of some interest to inquire as to what measures the Southland took to control disease. Was it as ready to defend itself against the economic

---

[7] Selling liquor to slaves was usually forbidden by law, though there was of course considerable "boot-legging." For court methods in dealing with violations thereof, see Catterall, *op. cit.*, II. 570, etc.

[8] John Spare, *Hunts Merchants Mag.*, XIII. 497 ff. *Cf.* Nott, *op. cit.*, for the fallacies in these figures.

[9] Robt. Jackson, . . . *Observations on the Intermitting Fever of America* (Phila., 1795), p. 21.

loss and human suffering thus occasioned, as it was against such financial losses as were threatened by tariff or abolition? The question can be answered, in large part, in terms of the development of medical science and a medical profession, since these agencies were the most obvious ones directed toward the social control of disease.

II

The early nineteenth century witnessed several scientific achievements which promised much for the health of the South. Most obvious was the introduction of vaccination, within a year or two of its discovery in England. Less generally known, but scarcely less significant, was the isolation of quinine from cinchona by French chemists in 1822,[10] as a result of which the employment of quinine sulphate in large doses was gradually introduced by Southern physicians during the ensuing decade. The new remedy was a more potent one than crude cinchona, and its use checked the high mortality occasioned by certain forms of malarial fever.[11] At the same time, an increasing consciousness of the prophylactic value of land drainage manifested itself in the towns, which consequently undertook measures most creditable to them in view of the small means at their disposal. Thus Savannah began in 1817, when it had a population of only about five thousand, to eliminate rice fields in its vicinity, and eventually appropriated two hundred thousand dollars to subsidize the planters involved in this abandonment of the "wet culture." Within a decade of the beginning of this work (undertaken at the behest of physicians), the mortality rate had dropped to less

[10] MM. Pelletier et Carenton, "Recherches Chimiques sur les Quinquinas," *Annales De Chimie Et De Physique*, 2 Ser., XV. 289 ff. (1822).

[11] *So. Med. Rep'ts.*, II. 347–350, 402–407, 450; *So. Med. and Surgical Jour.*, N. S. XVI. 796 (1860).

than half its former figure, apparently as a result of the drainage operations.[12]

Unfortunately, the partial control of small-pox and malaria which followed these developments was concomitant with the appearance of new and ominous diseases, notably cholera and yellow fever. Both attained pandemic proportions and invaded the Northern ports as well as the Southern, but yellow fever practically disappeared from the former after 1820, at the very time that some of the most serious Southern epidemics began. Yellow fever was largely restricted to the towns—for reasons now easily understood—and attacked chiefly the whites; [13] while cholera, more catholic in its taste, spread everywhere along commercial routes and drew no color line. The appearance of this "scourge of nations" on a plantation was a truly terrifying phenomenon. Overseers and slaves died within a few hours of the first appearance of symptoms. When cholera attacked Bishop Polk's Louisiana plantation in 1849, 220 of his 356 Negroes contracted the disease within two weeks' time, and 70 deaths ensued. The conditions obtaining during such a visitation can scarcely be imagined.[14]

Physicians the world over sought desperately but unavailingly for preventative or cure. Opium was approved as a remedy in Glasgow, and condemned in London; approved in Augusta and spurned in Savannah. One Southern practitioner, after trying sixteen different medicines and a half-dozen special procedures in addition, observed philosophically that "it has been well impressed on my mind that there is *no*

[12] Thos. Gamble, Jr., *Hist. of the Municipal Government of Savannah* (appended to mayor's annual rep't. for 1900), pp. 141–146; F. D. Lee and J. L. Agnew, *Historical Record of Savannah* (Sav., 1869), p. 186.

[13] This is indicated in mortality rates, as well as in contemporary accounts. The mortality rate of Savannah in 1854, when there was a yellow fever epidemic, was 9.79% for whites and only 3.43% for Negroes; W. Duncan, *Tabulated Mortality Record of . . . Savannah* (Sav., 1870), p. 36.

[14] W. A. Booth, "On the Cholera of Lafourche Interior," *So. Med. Rep'ts.*, I. 221. See also other reports on cholera, *ibid.*, I. 359 ff., 371 ff., etc.

one remedy for cholera." [15] Practical plantation observers did indeed declare that the exclusive use of pure rain water would prevent the disease; but here, as in other cases, empirical observation was in advance of the rational medicine of its day.

Meanwhile, yellow fever was even more baffling. At times it seemed a native product, at times an imported one. Now it seemed clearly contagious, again it was obviously non-contagious. Physicians who considered it non-contagious clamored for the removal of quarantines—and the merchants clamored with them. Others, backed by an hysterical public, demanded the traditional protection. Looking back, it is easy to find in insect transmission a key to all the apparently contradictory phenomena of yellow fever; but lacking that key, there was no problem more difficult of solution. [16]

Too much attention, however, should not be accorded the epidemics, for despite their spectacular and terrifying character, they were rarely so serious a menace as were the endemic ills—indeed they exerted a benign influence in arousing a demand for sanitary reform, which was more than the domesticated diseases could do. It follows that the routine treatment of ordinary illness was probably, from the social point of view, the most significant aspect of medical practice. [17]

[15] C. H. Stone, "Report on Epidemic Cholera in the Vicinity of Natchez," *ibid.*, p. 364.

[16] There are many accounts of the yellow fever epidemics; see G. D. Armstrong, *The Summer of Pestilence: A History of the Ravages of Yellow Fever in Norfolk, 1855* (Phila., 1856); *The Arnold Letters*, pp. 68 ff.; E. D. Fenner, "The Fevers of New Orleans," *So. Med. Rep'ts*. I. 106 ff., etc. A good picture of the confusion in medical opinion *re* this disease, is afforded in the long and tense debates in the Third National Quarantine and Sanitary Convention (N.Y., 1859); see *Proceedings of that body*, pp. 23–83.

[17] See M. P. Ravenel, "Endemic Diseases Versus Acute Epidemics," *Amer. Jour. of Pub. Health*, X. 761 ff. (1920); R. H. Shryock, "Origins and Significance of the Public Health Movement in the United States," *Annals of Medical History*, N.S., I. 645, 656 n. 12. The technical side of general practice, and its bases in contemporary pathology, therapeutics, etiology, etc., cannot be entered into here.

Now this cannot be measured entirely in terms of such information as was available to science. One must first ask: to what extent did Southern practitioners achieve a knowledge of such science as was then available; and, second, to what extent did they apply that knowledge *pro bono publico?*

III

Most regular American physicians, at the beginning of the nineteenth century, had been trained only by a preceptor, and there is no evidence that they read widely thereafter. The lack of urban cultural centers in the South retarded the development of medical schools and other professional institutions. In communities able to support several physicians, each viewed the others as so many competitors, and adopted at best an attitude of "armed neutrality" toward them.[18] Such conditions were not conducive to the rapid transit of medical culture from its center in Edinburgh to its periphery in Arkansas.

During the colonial period, as is well known, Americans occasionally went abroad for their medical training, and Charleston at one time boasted a larger number of such graduates than any other American town. It remained for the larger Northern cities, however, to take the next step necessary for the transfer of medical culture to this country; viz., to establish native schools, hospitals, societies, and journals. The consequence was that such Southerners as aspired to formal training were gradually diverted, after about 1800, from European institutions to the more conveniently located schools in Philadelphia, New York, and Lexington.[19] In like manner,

[18] *So. Jour. of Med. and Pharmacy,* I. 1 (1846); *So. Med. Rep'ts.,* II. 458.

[19] Of 144 men graduating from the Medical School of the University of Pennsylvania in 1838—a year taken at random—more than half were Southerners. There were 40 Virginians in contrast to 21 Pennsylvanians; *Amer. Jour. of the Med. Sciences,* XXII. 259–263 (1838). See also *So. Med. and Surg. Jour.,* N. S., II. 383 (1846).

the first cities named partially replaced foreign centers in the manufacture of medical supplies for the Southern trade. It was obvious that medical dependence on the North was an established fact by 1830.

Certain influences, however, were destined to arouse a protest against this dependence within a decade. The continued growth of some six or eight Southern cities promoted a corresponding growth of professional consciousness therein. Hospitals were established,[20] and local medical societies organized—once the jealousies of the "small town" practitioner could be partially overcome. Thus the "Georgia Medical Society" of Savannah was founded as early as 1804, and most Southern cities boasted such organizations by 1830. State societies, promoted by the local bodies, appeared about two decades later, but received a rather uncertain support from the profession at large. Meanwhile, a number of able physicians in Augusta had made in 1836 the first formal attempt to organize a national medical association; only to have the move thwarted (they claimed) by the indifference or opposition of the University of Pennsylvania.[21] When the plan was again taken up by the New York State Medical Society (1846), Southern leaders coöperated in the organization and early administration of the American Medical Association.

Professional leaders in the larger Southern towns were naturally the first to envisage a sectional medical culture sufficiently mature to provide its own training centers. They had found that Northern or foreign training had not entirely prepared them for the Southern scene. Southern diseases had their peculiarities, apparently unknown to Yankee professors —and so had Southern Negroes! Under these circumstances

---

[20] The early history of the largest such institution in the ante-bellum South, the Charity Hospital of New Orleans, is given in the *New Orleans Med. Jour.*, I. 72–77 (1844).

[21] *So. Med. and Surg. Jour.*, I. 220 (1836).

the native professional school, treating of native conditions, seemed to be indicated.[22] It remained for urban medical groups to risk the venture. Charleston, the oldest scientific center in the South, was appropriately enough the site of its first medical school—the "Medical College of the State of South Carolina," established in 1823. At almost the same time, a Medical Department was organized at the University of Virginia. Similar institutions were founded during the next decade at Augusta (1832), New Orleans (1835), and Richmond (1838). These pioneer colleges adopted the standards which then obtained among the better Northern schools (involving a four or five months' course of lectures plus preceptorial requirements) and compared favorably with most of the older institutions. They eventually received some assistance from state or local governments, and steadily increased their enrollments until 1861.[23]

No sooner had a faculty organized a college than it began looking about for ways and means to finance a journal. This was quite logically the next step in the establishment of an indigenous scientific culture,[24] for a journal could represent the school and, at the same time, serve as a medium for professional exchange over a large area. The first such periodical printed south of the border states was the *Southern Journal of Medicine and Surgery*, established by Dr. Milton Antony at Augusta in 1836, discontinued at his death in '39, and reëstablished in '45. In the latter year Dr. E. D. Fenner

[22] Paul Eve, E. D. Fenner, and Samuel Cartwright were the leading advocates for Southern training; see *So. Med. Rep'ts.*, I. 354, II. 423, *New Orleans Med. and Surg. Jour.*, II. 731 (1846).

[23] The risks ventured and success attained are well illustrated in the case of the New Orleans college; see *So. Med. Rep'ts.*, I. 461–463. Note also *So. Med. and Surg. Jour.*, II. 703, III. 2, 3 (1837, 38); *Savannah Med. Jour.*, II. 56 (1860), etc.

[24] This phrase is used advisedly, as even at this late date the versatile type of physician was likely to be the leading local exponent of the natural sciences in general. This interesting phase of medical history cannot be entered into here.

founded the *New Orleans Medical Journal,* and shortly thereafter a Charleston group launched the *Southern Journal of Medicine and Pharmacy.* All were well edited and compared favorably with most of the Northern publications. They were followed, during the fifties, by acceptable journals at Nashville (1851), Richmond (1851), Savannah (1859), and, finally, by the short-lived *Confederate States Medical and Surgical Reporter*—published in the capital of the Confederacy.

Through the medium of their journals, the Southern faculties increasingly stressed the need for local training; and as the state medical societies began to publish their transactions, the same propaganda appeared therein. This naturally aroused some anxiety in the Northern schools, whence came occasional counter-blasts to the effect that Southern faculties were exploiting sectional feeling simply in order to increase the enrollment of their own schools. Both Paul Eve and Cartwright became involved in controversies with Northern professors concerning the relative merit of the Southern institutions.[25] It is important to note that such friction possessed more than a purely professional significance.[26] While it is true that the development of medical institutions in the South was in large part simply a phase of cultural development going on throughout the nation, it was also characterized by considerable sectional consciousness. The very period of this medical development, 1820–1860, was also a time of increasing sectional tension all along the line; a tension which led in the

[25] B. B. Mitchell, "Southern Versus Northern Practice," *The Medical Examiner,* N. S., IV. 591 ff. (Phila., 1848); *New Orleans Med. Jour.,* III. 259 ff. (1846). It should be remembered, of course, that cordial relations existed between some Northern and Southern leaders; see, e.g. *The Arnold Letters, passim.*

[26] It is a curious fact that, after all their thunder, Southern faculties never introduced any courses dealing especially with Southern diseases or the Negroes; see *Savannah Med. Jour.,* II. 61 (1860).

South to a growing desire for cultural,[27] as well as for economic and (eventually) political independence of the North. Southern physicians therefore felt a sort of patriotic obligation to improve their guild and render it self-sustaining. Even their emphasis on the peculiarities of Negro diseases was associated with an emphasis upon the inherent biological distinctions between the races,[28] and this in turn was an integral part of the whole pro-slavery argument.

Southern leaders were not able, perhaps did not desire, to divert *all* Southern students from the Yankee schools. The years immediately preceding the Civil War, therefore, found these students representing—in certain cases—the largest Southern groups resident in Northern communities. As sectional feeling approached the breaking point, their presence became the occasion for various expressions of animosity. In Philadelphia there had been rumblings of this sort as early as 1837, but the storm broke in 1860, when some three hundred medical students left that city in a body for Richmond.[29]

[27] Note, e.g., such verse as the following; taken from *Georgia Illustrated* (Penfield, Ga., 1841):

> Sons of the South, whose hearts beat high,
>   With generous pride and aim
> To make your land and birthplace vie
>   With any land in fame.
> While justly ye extoll the skies,
>   Your clime and fertile land,
> The brightness of your maidens' eyes,
>   Their voices soft and bland . . .
> While these ye boast and proudly dare
>   The world their peers to show,
> Are ye content with humble share
>   Of gifts from mind, which flow? . . .
> Sons of the South! shall it be said
>   Ye prize not mental store?
> Oh! bid the fires of Genius spread
>   Our sunny region o'er.

[28] See, e.g., J. C. Nott and G. R. Gliddon, *Types of Mankind*, etc. (Phila. 1854); J. H. Van Evrie, *Negroes and Negro Slavery* (New York, 1853). The former was edited by physicians.

[29] *So. Med. and Surg. Jour.,* N. S., XVI. 236 (1860).

Similar friction, in which no doubt the students played their part, developed in New York. In this connection, the editor of the New York *Sun* revealed the opinion of these men entertained in some quarters. "The Southern medical student," he observed kindly, "is well known in the neighborhood of 13th St., . . . & 4th Ave. He is a long-haired, lantern-jawed, verdant youth, afflicted with chronic salivation and inveterate profanity. Reared in the semi-savage solitude of a remote plantation, and deriving his ideas of morals, grammar, and behavior from his negro nurse and picaninny playmates, he becomes in New York a puzzle to professors, a terror to landladies, and a munificent patron of grogshops. Having finished his so-called course of study . . . he returns to his native wilds to commence practice on a pretentious stock of medical ignorance, calomel, and quinine. Next to his taste for tobacco and grog comes his taste for Disunion. Ignorant of law . . . his stock of political ideas consists wholly of hatred of the people to whom he is obliged to come for instruction." In noting this interesting tribute, the *Nashville Medical and Surgical Journal* inquired of "the young gentlemen of the South" how they "liked this picture." [30] It is regrettable that their reply is not at hand.

One of the most interesting sectional controversies within the medical profession was that precipitated by Oliver Wendell Holmes when, in an interesting report to the American Medical Association in 1848, he referred to "the efflorescence of scientific enthusiasm on the banks of the Mississippi and Missouri," and to "inferior schools wrongly located" in these regions.[31] The discussion eventually descended to remarks on "Boston notions," Dr. Holmes' sophomoric style, and to a polite suggestion by the latter that Southern editors would do well to learn their own language.

[30] *Savannah Med. Jour.,* II. 369, 370 (1861).
[31] The report is given in the *A.M.A. Trans.,* I. 283–288.

There was, unfortunately, some truth in Dr. Holmes' "Boston notions." There were, by 1848, some "inferior schools wrongly located"—though they were not confined to any one section. What was worse, the number increased rapidly during the 'fifties. What was still worse, the lowering of educational standards in such colleges was associated with other influences making for a general demoralization of medical practice. The rapid extension of the Southern frontier after 1815 had opened up areas in which, as in any new country, the popular status of culture in general, and of medical science in particular, was inevitably low. Frontier farmers—Jacksonian Democrats—were not appreciative of professional training, and consequently were not inclined to make nice distinctions between regular and irregular practitioners. Moreover, a growing suspicion that the orthodox physicians were ineffective began to manifest itself even among the educated classes. At the same time the high disease rate noted, plus the ordinary needs of a growing population, created a great demand for doctors of some sort. These conditions resulted in an increasing patronage accorded to quackery,[32] and such new sects as homeopathy, Thomsonianism, and hydropathy, and in the gradual abandonment of practically all state licensing restrictions.[33]

Everyone was allowed to practice medicine by 1850, and it was only mild exaggeration to say that everyone did! Planters, housewives, overseers, pharmacists, sectarians, quacks—all had a hand in the game. Here and there a "doctress" without formal training anticipated and perhaps prepared the way for

[32] Cartwright's study of quackery in Natchez convinced him that it was the cause of more deaths there than were all diseases put together! *So. Med. and Surg. Jour.*, N. S., IV. 767 (1848). See also his "Remarks on Statistical Medicine, Contrasting the Result of the Empirical with the Regular Practice of Physic," *Amer. Jour. of the Med. Sciences*, N. S., I. 271–275 (1841).

[33] *New York State Med. Soc. Proceeds.*, 1844, *passim*.

the later women physicians.[34] Such practice was not necessarily all bad. Most lay dabbling, however, depended at best upon the family medical manuals, and, at worst, upon magic and sheer humbug. Even Negro slaves practiced in one way or another, and were in some cases consulted by the whites and allowed to give all their time to their profession.[35] The following advertisement for patients, written by a Negro in 1860, is suggestive of a type of practice which survives in the work of Negro mid-wives to the present day:

> T. Edwards is naturally a Doctor—having a gift from the Lord. My mother was her mother's seventh daughter, and I am her seventh son . . . I am a seven months' child, and walked seven months after I was born, and have shed my teeth seven times.[36]

Such professional qualifications must, in certain circles, have proved irresistible.

IV

In this connection, it should be observed that the medical care of Negro slaves was perhaps the most distinctive phase of Southern practice. The slaves were the only group of poor workers in whose health their employers had a direct property interest, and for whom they felt a direct personal responsibility; and for these reasons they sometimes received more care than did Southern "poor whites" or Northern laborers. It was not unknown for a white mistress to nurse slave babies so ill

---

[34] Catterall, *Judicial Cases*, II. 531, 576. The reaction of the Southern newspapers to the first regular women physicians was generally favorable. Even some doctors adopted a friendly attitude; see *Savannah Med. Jour.*, II. 372 ff. (1860).

[35] Catterall, *op. cit.*, II. 43, 144, 414, 520, 521. The Tennessee Court decided, 1844, that slaves should not practice—not out of fear for patients, but from fear such doctors might foment insurrections.

[36] *Cf.* C. C. Van Blarcom, "Rat Pie: Black Midwives and Black Magic," *Harpers Mag.*, CLX, 322–332 (Feb., 1930).

with diphtheria that their own mothers feared to touch them. On some of the better plantations a carefully devised regimen and sanitary police were provided, as well as attendance by a regular physician.[37] The leading practitioners were sometimes so employed, but more usually the beginners—sometimes upon a contract basis.[38] Thus the young Southern physician found in slavery a means to an early start; while at the same time, the slaves found in the system a sort of health insurance. Hence emancipation injured the practice of many doctors, and the health of many ex-slaves, since the former could not afford to attend a poor Negro, once he had become "nobody's nigger but his own." [39]

Some evidence that this would be the case was collected,

[37] See, e.g., *De Bow's Review*, XXII. 38–44, as reprinted in J. S. Bassett, *The Plantation Overseer* (Northampton, 1925), pp. 28, 29.

[38] Contract practice was fairly common, at this time, in the case of the younger or less successful men, but was condemned by the leaders as cheap and unprofessional. The latter were almost as much concerned then over low fees (e.g., 25 or 50 cents a visit) as laymen are today over high charges. Average annual incomes for country practitioners in Alabama were reported as about one thousand dollars; for those in a small town, two thousand dollars (*So. Med. Rep'ts.*, I. 257). The itemized plantation bills of prominent physicians, however, do not seem so low. Thus Dr. Tomlinson Fort of Milledgeville received from Col. F. Carter, for services on the latter's place in Georgia, such amounts as the following:

1839	Ap. 1	N.M.	Visit 4 miles, 5.00, prescription.	$ 6.00
			Negroes and son, med. and prescrip-	
	" 22		tion.	2.00
	May 1		Negro child med.	1.00
	" 22	N.M.	Visit 4 miles 5.00. med, for gonor-	
			rhea	15.00
1841	Ap. 7	N.	Visit 4 mi. & opg abcess	6.00
	May 13		Visit 4 miles in rain & med	7.00
	June 24		Visit noct. 4 mi	8.00

etc. etc. (Bills in possession of Dr. R. B. Flanders, of New York University. Differences in purchasing power are to be kept in mind.)

[39] Except, of course, as part of his charity work. For contemporary comment on post-emancipation suffering among Negroes, see *The Arnold Letters*, pp. 129–131. A survey of the whole subject is given in F. L. Hoffman, *Race Traits and Tendencies of the American Negro* (Pubs. Amer. Econom. Asso., XI), 33 ff.

even before emancipation, by means of a comparison of the free Negro and slave Negro mortality rates. Nott claimed that the free Negro mortality in Northern cities was two to three times that of slaves in Charleston, remarking that "freedom and climate, combined in Boston, are far more destructive to the negro than slavery and Asiatic cholera at the South." Moreover, he found that in Baltimore (where the climatic factor was a constant) the free Negro death rate was more than twice that of the slaves.[40] Nott, however, was not on the reading lists of abolitionists.

The owner's concern for the health of his property expressed itself dramatically in times of epidemics, when the whole plantation personnel might be moved to a more salubrious location, even at the expense of the year's crop. It is easy to understand this, when it is recalled that the loss from slave deaths in one cholera epidemic in Louisiana alone (1833) was estimated at four million dollars! [41] Again, when extra-hazardous work was to be done, as ditch-digging in a malarial region, Irish laborers were sometimes employed to save the slaves.[42] Traders, as well as permanent owners, showed concern for their property in times of special danger, and would take their gangs to the pines to avoid the same. Incidentally, the domestic slave trade—like the foreign before it—was a factor in the spread of disease. Thus Natchez, a trading center, witnessed an almost annual introduction of contagious diseases *via* the gangs brought in for sale.[43]

The property right in slave patients occasionally placed physicians in a peculiar legal position; as when one was sued

---

[40] "Health and Longevity in the Southern Sea Ports," *So. Jour. of Med. and Pharmacy.* II. 138 (1847). See also Lemuel Shattuck's interesting notes on the Negro in Boston; "On the Vital Statistics of Boston," *Amer. Jour. of the Med. Sciences*, N. S., I. 371, 377 (1841).

[41] *Niles Register*, XLV. 84.

[42] Phillips, *Life and Labor in the Old South*, pp. 186, 187.

[43] *So. Med. and Surg. Jour.*, N. S., IV. 767.

by a planter for the loss of a slave committed to his care. It also seems strange, from our present point of view, that a master might order medical procedure, such as an operation, without regard to the wishes of a slave patient.[44] Last, but not least curious, was the fact that a perversion of the property interest actually might prevent a sick slave from receiving medical attention, whenever an indifferent owner was convinced the case was hopeless.[45]

This last situation, rare though it was, suggests the other side of the story—there were disadvantages in slavery as a system of health insurance. After all, the large plantation with a well-organized medical régime was an exceptional institution, save in certain rich areas. On the ordinary place the master, mistress, or overseer was likely to look after all but the obviously serious cases among their people. This policy was dictated by considerations of economy if for no other reason— it was natural for an overseer to report that he sent for a doctor "only when it was indispensably necessary." Physicians were therefore less likely to be called in to see Negroes, than for whites in the same region.[46] Obstetrical cases were usually handled by ignorant Negro mid-wives, and the high incidence of uterine diseases among slave women, and of tetanus among their newborn, were doubtless the results of this system.[47] Miscarriages were reported as relatively frequent among Negro women, as a result of overwork, or—as some planters

[44] Catterall, *Judicial Cases,* I. 373, 404, 441.

[45] *Ibid.,* II. 108.

[46] *Ibid.,* II, 460; *So. Med. Rep'ts.,* I. 336 ff. Cartwright referred to "the practice among three millions of people [Negroes] that the overseers have mostly got"; *So. Med. Rep'ts.,* II. 423.

[47] *Trismus Nascentium* was reported as occurring "with fearful frequency" among the Negroes of the Gulf states, but as being very rare among the whites, *So. Med. and Surg. Jour.,* N.S., II. 432, 433. See also E. M. Pendleton's essays, "On the Susceptibility of the Caucasian and African Races to the Different Classes of Disease," *So. Med. and Surg. Jour.,* Nov., 1849, and ". . . the Diseases of Middle Georgia," *So. Med. Rep'ts.,* I. 336 ff.

believed—of a frequent resort to criminal abortion.[48] "A vast proportion of negro babies die within ten days after birth," observed the editor of an Alabama agricultural journal, who went on to estimate that their death rate was about double that of white infants in his region.[49]

The Negro children who survived were often suckled by hurried or overheated mothers from the fields, were more or less filthy, and were commonly infected with intestinal parasites of one sort or another. Adult slaves were subject to neglect, involving at times inadequate clothing, filth, and unhealthy diet, over-heavy burdens, etc. It is a suggestive fact that hernia was reported from widely separated regions, as being unusually common among slaves.[50] Some of the bad conditions obtaining among Negroes, to be sure, may be ascribed to their own "laziness" or superstition, while mere ignorance was also a factor among both men and masters. Yet the net result, whatever the causes, was often an unhappy one. In a word, the *a priori* argument for slave health, in terms of a property interest, has only a partial validity,—men have been known to neglect even their livestock.

V

Enough has now been said of the shortcomings of medical work among both the blacks and whites. The picture of Southern practice in general would be incomplete, after the manner of modern fiction, were no mention made of the more pleasing aspects of the story. It has been noted that many Americans of this period had small regard for regular practi-

[48] *Ibid.*, p. 338.

[49] Rural mortality rates were rarely kept for this period, though county records were occasionally compiled (e.g., in the county census report of Georgia for 1860); hence the comparative rural rates for whites and Negroes are not available. Urban rates were usually higher for whites, but there were exceptions to this, as in the case of Charleston after 1840. See Hoffman, *op. cit.*, pp. 53, 54.

[50] See *The Arnold Letters*, p. 13.

tioners, but it should be added that many others continued to have such faith in their physicians as is rare in our own times. If this faith was at times misplaced, it should at least be recalled that there were other than scientific grounds for confidence. When the Southern physician called on his patient, the chances were that he came some distance, that he came willingly whenever he was called, and that he was welcomed upon arrival as the old friend and father-confessor of the household. In a word, he belonged to that now declining species, the "family doctor." Such men worked hard at their practice, and sometimes harder to collect their bills from such as could afford to pay them.[51] Richard Arnold, a successful city practitioner, wrote in 1849 that, besides about sixty-five ward patients, "the average of my private patients in the late summer and fall months is generally between thirty and forty and to get through with these . . . I am going the rounds from sunrise to nine or ten o'clock at night . . . it is frequently necessary to see a patient three or four times a day." Again he observed: "It runs me almost crazy to think that with hundreds upon hundreds due me professionally I find the greatest difficulty in raising a simple fifty dollars." [52]

In the absence of any well organized system of poor relief, much of the burden of charity practice fell directly on the shoulders of the physicians. It was estimated in 1861 that in one fairly prosperous Georgia county alone, the doctors gave away annually about thirty thousand dollars' worth of quinine.[53] While then, as now, they must have passed such

[51] The doctor's bill was usually the last one paid. Dr. Fort's bill to Col. Carter for 1839 (noted above) totaled $73.75. Under this figure was added later the suggestive statement: "8 years Int. 8% 47.20"!

[52] *The Arnold Letters*, pp. 21, 170, 171.

[53] The State courts were directed by law to look after such poor, and a tax levied for that purpose, but nothing was done about it—hence public opinion expected the doctors to supply free medicine as well as free service; *So. Med. and Surg. Jour.*, N.S., XVII. 347, 348 (1861). It will be noted in this connection that the differentiation between physician and

expenses on in higher charges to paying patients, the fact remains that this was a poorly adjusted system that might work hardships upon an individual physician, as well as upon those who met their bills.

One of life's little ironies for the doctor, moreover, was the fact that it was often in this charitable work that he ran the greatest personal risk from contagion. This risk was very real, especially in times of epidemics, and the mortality among doctors was high. When yellow fever attacked Savannah in 1854, that city had a population of about eighteen thousand, including from twenty-five to thirty regular physicians. Within a few weeks no less than ten of the latter had succumbed to "the yellow monster." [54]

In view of all these circumstances, it is small wonder that some good people maintained faith in the family doctor, whatever the latter's scientific limitations. It is probably a legitimate assumption, moreover, that the development of Southern medical institutions was related as both cause and effect to some improvement in even the scientific status of Southern practitioners. Further evidence to this effect may be found in the participation by Southern men in the work of medical research and experimentation, characteristic of the more critical spirit manifested in medical science during this period. Indeed, the amount of original work achieved by Southern physicians, in view of their relative isolation, was truly remarkable. One has only to recall the place held in American medical history by such men as McDowell, Sims,

---

pharmacist, so long established in Europe, was very imperfect in the United States of 1860. County practitioners still performed the functions of physician, pharmacist, and even dentist, and the states required nothing in the way of standards of the druggists in the towns. On Southern pharmacy see *So. Jour. of Med. and Pharmacy,* I. 308 (1846), and the *New Orleans Med. and Surg. Jour.,* II. 728 (1846). The history of dentistry, of veterinary medicine, and of nursing, cannot be entered into within the limits of this paper.

[54] See files of the Savannah *Republican,* Aug. 15 to Oct. 15, 1854.

Nott, Drake, and Crawford W. Long, in order to make this point clear.[55] It is not exaggerating to say that despite all the demoralizing influences noted above, the Southern medical profession faced a fairly promising future at the end of the ante-bellum period.

Then in 1861 came the tragedy of civil war, and with it the diversion of medical activity to the field. The story of the Confederate medical service is still worthy of study. The end of the war saw Southern medical culture necessarily involved in the general disaster. Defeat meant poverty, and poverty meant that professional income fell, schools closed or stagnated, journals discontinued. In medicine, as in other phases of life, the South had to rebuild as best it could.[56] Only after a generation had passed, and with the advent of a new prosperity, did there come a renaissance in Southern medicine.

[55] Interesting comment on the original work of Southern physicians is found in J. Marion Sims' "Normal Ovariotomy—Battey's Operation," *North Carolina Med. Jour.*, I. 26–28 (1878). See also W. A. Lewis, "The History of Medicine in the South," *Va. Med. Monthly*, XLVIII. 655–660 (1922); E. Souchon, "Original Contributions of America to Medical Sciences," *Trans. Amer. Surg. Asso.*, XXXV. 165–171 (1917).

[56] See G. H. Tichenor, "Medicine During the Reconstruction Period, 1865–1900, in the South; Terrible Lessons," *Western Medical Times*, XLI. 339–343 (1922).

III

American Indifference
to Basic Science
during the Nineteenth Century *

The general indifference to basic research displayed in the United States during the greater part of the nineteenth century, is a significant phenomenon in the history of modern science. In contrast, the American record in applied science—in technology, inventions, surgical practice—was a distinguished one. This technological achievement was important. It exercised a world influence, and its merit should not be underestimated by assumptions about the superiority of "pure science" per se. It is an even more serious mistake, however, to assume the superiority of applied science; and this is what Americans tended to do—almost unconsciously—during the past century. This error was recognized by American scientists themselves when, from time to time, they urged that more heed should be given to fundamental investigations.[1]

If the lag in basic research in the United States could be ascribed simply to a lack of facilities in a new country, any

* Reprinted from *Archives Internationales d'Histoire des Sciences*, No. 5 (1948)—by permission.
[1] This appeal was still being made at the end of the century. See, e.g., William Pepper, *Higher Medical Education*, Lippincott, Philadelphia, 1894, pp. 1 ff.

further analysis of the phenomenon would be of little interest. No one expects a relatively poor and isolated people to contribute much to the arts and sciences. This was the situation of various colonial populations during recent times; but the Americans had risen above this level even before the end of the eighteenth century. As early as 1760, for example, Philadelphia had become one of the chief centers of the Enlightenment in the English-speaking world.[2]

A century later, by 1860, the United States had attained a population of over thirty millions and wealth was accumulating from the exploitation of vast natural resources. Earlier European enthusiasm for the American experiment in "democracy" was now tempered by realistic criticisms of the crudity or naïveté of American society. But it is misleading to think of the United States, at midcentury, as a "new," primitive, or unsophisticated country in any ordinary sense of those terms. It possessed the basic conditions and facilities usually considered essential to cultural activity. Large cities, wealth, learned institutions, intellectual freedom, and an optimistic faith in "progress"—all these were available. Close cultural contacts had long been maintained with both Britain and France, while, at the same time, nationalistic feeling demanded national originality.[3] In certain fields, notably in literature, the results were all that might have been anticipated. The generation which produced Emerson, Whitman, and Poe was capable of intellectual activity of a high order.

Yet, in science, the story was a far different one. None of the American cities had become research centers in the sense

---

[2] Carl and Jessica Bridenbaugh, *Rebels and Gentlemen: Philadelphia in The Age of Franklin,* Reynal and Hitchcock, New York, 1942, pp. 361 ff.

[3] The demand for national originality was stimulated by the Revolution, and later by British criticisms, and led to some exaggerated claims concerning national achievements. See Merle Curti, *The Growth of American Thought,* Harper and Brothers, New York, 1943, pp. 245 ff.

that were London, Paris, and Berlin, and few individuals were devoted primarily to research careers. The exceptions, such as Joseph Henry in physics and Joseph Leidy in biology, only proved the rule. Here, then, was a country well equipped to pursue basic investigations; but which actually neglected them, and excelled only in their applications. An analysis of this paradox may throw some light upon the influence which society exerts upon science.

It has been suggested that Americans found it so easy to borrow science from abroad that they felt no need to provide it for themselves. Tocqueville, in 1835, advanced this as one of the factors explaining the failure of Americans to cultivate what he termed "theoretical" science. "I am convinced," he wrote, "that if the Americans had been alone in the world . . . they would not have been slow to discover that progress cannot long be made in the application of the sciences without cultivating the theory of them. . . ." This conjecture, in the nature of the case, cannot be proved or disproved; but Tocqueville himself went on to note the danger that in a too "close adherence to mere applications, principles would be lost sight of, and when the principles were wholly forgotten, the methods derived from them would be ill pursued." He even cited isolated Chinese civilization, "absorbed in productive industry," as an actual instance of this outcome.[4] One might have feared a similar result, if America had been isolated. In any case, the mere availability of European theoretical science cannot, in itself, explain American indifference to its cultivation. Over and over again, in Europe, the availability of more advanced, basic science in one country served as a stimulus— rather than as a deterrent—to its cultivation in another. There must have been other factors in American civilization which explained the difference in the American reaction.

[4] Alexis De Tocqueville, *Democracy in America,* translated by Henry Reeve, D. Appleton, New York, II, 1904, p. 518.

A second thesis, commonly held, is that Americans were necessarily preoccupied with "subduing Nature" or "conquering a continent." [5] They were so busy laying the material bases of civilization that they had little time or interest left for cultural matters. Unfortunately, "subduing Nature" is a vague phrase. If it implies that most men were actually engaged in clearing a wilderness or building homes, the thesis is absurd except for the times and places of original settlement. A variation on this theme is the assertion that since Americans were the descendants of immigrants and pioneers, they all inherited the attitudes of immigrants and pioneers—with a resulting neglect of cultural activities. To put it more definitely: it may be that the primitive conditions of early settlement left some imprint upon later states of mind. Having once turned, necessarily, to the mother lands for science and art, the people of the United States may have formed a habit of dependence which persisted into years of wealth and maturity. It is difficult to generalize about this, since some Americans always showed an exaggerated awe for things European, while others displayed an equally exaggerated and even boastful independence. The inherited awe did lead at times to slavish imitation in the arts and sciences, but this did not prevent real achievement in certain aspects of culture. It is difficult to see why science should have been the peculiar victim of a persisting colonial state of mind.

If the phrase "conquering a continent" implies only that most Americans were busy exploiting natural resources, one wonders why they *were* so preoccupied? The mere existence of these resources did not necessarily lead to such activities among European settlers, as is evident from the very different history of minority groups of French peasants in Quebec and of German peasants in Pennsylvania. Various qualities which

[5] See, e.g., Henry B. Parkes, *The American Experience*, Alfred A. Knopf, New York, 1947, pp. 9 ff.

the dominating British peoples brought with them—puritanism, capitalistic acquisitiveness, relatively free attitudes and institutions—all interacted with the environment to produce social democracy and the desire of every man to "get ahead" in a material way. From this situation sprang the apparent materialism, the vulgarization, and the "commercial mindedness" which European travelers noted and which many a native critic deplored.

Tocqueville, probably the ablest foreign observer, believed that the combination of democracy and of economic opportunities inevitably led to a neglect of theoretical science and to a cultivation of technology. The masses, favored by equalitarian opportunities, sought in science only the immediate means to exploiting natural wealth in the interest of their own comfort. On the other hand, there was no class in a democratic society which possessed either the tradition or the leisure to cultivate the more contemplative, theoretical aspects of science. "In aristocratic ages," declared the French observer, "science is more particularly called upon to furnish gratification to the mind; in democracies to the body." He believed, nevertheless, that basic science would emerge in the United States and in other democracies, if the "constituted authorities" would deliberately encourage those individuals who were inclined to it. Technology, meanwhile, would take care of itself.[6]

Tocqueville's analysis of the American situation remains one of the most valid which has been provided. Subsequent experience suggests, however, that it is incomplete in some respects and calls for refinement in others. His view that intellectual interests in general, as well as science in particular, were inhibited by American conditions, cannot be entirely reconciled with the record. Theology had flourished in colonial New England, reaching a high point in Jonathan

---

[6] Tocqueville, *op. cit.*, pp. 524 ff.

Edwards.[7] Even basic science had flourished in the Philadelphia of 1750, reaching its high point in Franklin.[8] And soon after Tocqueville wrote, there ensued the literary "flowering" of the Emerson–Poe–Whitman era. Tocqueville offers no explanation of the peculiar neglect of basic science in the nineteenth century. Some refinement of certain of his categories, such as those of "classes," "the multitude," and "utility," may assist in explaining this neglect in further discussion below.

A third thesis relates inertia in the natural sciences to the clerical control of colleges and universities. Such control continued longer in American institutions than it did in outstanding Continental universities. And it was only after about 1875, when the direct influence of the Protestant churches upon universities was declining, that there was a marked increase in the latter's scientific activities. But this sequence does not prove that the churches had discouraged research up to that time. Science had flourished in a Protestant environment during the sixteenth and seventeenth centuries in Europe,[9] and this tradition was maintained to some degree in American colleges during the ensuing period.[10] After about 1780, Protestant clergy in the United States did display some fear of science because of the spread of deism and unitarianism. The subsequent religious "revivals" produced an orthodox atmosphere in the colleges which was hostile to "free thinkers." French medicine of 1840 was occasionally condemned as materialistic, and the opposition to "Darwinism" after 1860 is well known.

[7] See Perry Miller, *The New England Mind,* Macmillan, New York, 1939.

[8] See I. Bernard Cohen, "How Practical Was Benjamin Franklin's Science?" *Pennsylvania Magazine of History and Biography* (Philadelphia), vol. 69, Oct. 1945, p. 284.

[9] Jean Pelseneer, "L'Origine Protestante de la Science Moderne," *Lychnos* (Uppsala), 1946–1947, pp. 246–248.

[10] Theodore Hornberger, *Scientific Thought in the American Colleges, 1638–1800,* University of Texas Press, Austin, 1945, pp. 80 ff.

But there is little evidence that the churches directly opposed scientific work in the better schools of this period. Professional opportunities were doubtless best for scientists who were sympathetic with, or at least not hostile to, the prevailing forms of Christianity; but there were many such men who could have pursued basic research without fear of ecclesiastical opposition. The view that science revealed the glory of God persisted, and resulted in some encouragement of science teaching in even the most orthodox circles. Moreover, independent institutes and academies in the larger cities functioned in an entirely secular environment. Even if some clergymen distrusted science, it must be remembered that there was no state church in the United States and that there was therefore no common ecclesiastical policy. In the presence of various denominations and their rival institutions, there was room for liberalism in certain schools if this was denied in others.

One concludes that religious enthusiasms inhibited science only in a rather negative and indirect manner. The quasi-religious influence of German idealism enabled some science professors to hide their lack of originality behind a sonorous *Naturphilosophie*. But not until about 1890 did an extreme form of philosophical idealism, "Christian Science," become a popular cult which openly opposed scientific interests. Meanwhile, the churches indirectly inhibited the support of science by focusing public interest on religious issues and by attracting the more able men into clerical careers. At Yale College in 1850, for example, it was found that the most promising graduates who entered the professions chose theology or law in preference to medicine.[11] Philanthropy, as well as personnel, flowed into ecclesiastical channels. As late as 1891, it was openly stated that American theological schools possessed a total endowment of $18,000,000; whereas medical schools

---

[11] *Transactions,* American Medical Association, vol. 4, 1851, p. 409.

could boast of only \$500,000.[12] The endowment of departments or institutes of the physical sciences at this time was also negligible. Such contrasts, however, were the result rather than the cause of the greater prestige of religious interests.

One step removed from religious influence was the operation of a moral attitude which, after 1800, was most marked among the Anglo-Saxon peoples. This was the opposition to the dissection of the human body. How far this expressed traditional moral feeling, and to what extent it reflected a growing Victorian prudishness, is difficult to say. The inhibiting influence of this attitude was limited to the medical field; but therein it was of real significance, because it prevented autopsies at the very time when studies in pathologic anatomy were essential to the whole advance of basic medical science. Popular feeling also discouraged the training of physicians for clinical research, because medical students were denied access to hospital wards. This denial apparently resulted from equalitarian feeling for the rights of the poor, who must not be embarrassed as the mere subjects of student observations. Somewhat akin to the opposition to dissections was the antivivisection movement of the later nineteenth century, which handicapped the biological sciences and was also primarily an Anglo-Saxon phenomenon. This dangerous type of sentimentality is still much alive in the United States today.[13]

Quasi-moral or prudish attitudes indirectly handicapped certain other types of research in the United States, such as that on venereal disease.[14] But since influences of this sort

[12] G. M. Gould, "The Duty of the Community to Medical Science," *Bulletin,* The American Academy of Medicine, vol. I, Aug. 1893, p. 331.
[13] Richard H. Shryock, *American Medical Research: Past and Present,* Commonwealth Fund, New York, 1947, pp. 20, 61, 68.
[14] Shryock, "Freedom and Interference in Medicine," *Annals,* The American Academy of Political and Social Science (Philadelphia), vol. 200, 1938, p. 44.

related only to special aspects of medical science, they cannot account for the neglect of basic science in general.

A clue to the explanation of this larger phenomenon, however, is finally provided in the contrast noted at the start; that is, in the difference between American attitudes toward pure and applied science. This implies that utility was highly appreciated, but that there was little interest in abstract studies offering no promise of immediate usefulness. In this contrast one has a formula which clarifies the entire situation. It explains why national patent law was so planned as to encourage originality among inventors, and why successful men of this type—from Robert Fulton to Thomas A. Edison —were so highly esteemed. It also explains the aid granted to geologic surveys and to agricultural studies, by federal and state governments which would do almost nothing to assist research in astronomy, mathematical physics, or physiology. A clear test of governmental attitudes was afforded by the persistent refusal of Congress to support national scientific organizations, such as the National Institution in Washington (1840–1847); and it was only through the gift of an English-man that the Smithsonian Institution was finally established there.[15]

Private philanthropy was no more inclined to aid basic science than was government. When hospitals were subsidized, this was to provide for the sick poor; when universities were endowed, this was for the education of youth. Such research as was done in these institutions was incidental to their main functions. Professors in the arts colleges—including scientists—were mildly esteemed as teachers, but viewed otherwise as rather useless and "impractical" persons. Neither the salary nor the prestige accorded "M. le professeur" or the

[15] Madge E. Picard, "Government and Science in the United States: Historical Backgrounds," *Journal of the History of Medicine* (New York), vol. 1, April 1946, p. 254.

"Herr Doctor Professor" in Europe were granted to his American colleagues. Willard Gibbs, the greatest mathematical physicist in the United States, taught for years at Yale without receiving any salary whatever. Since "practical" success was apt to be measured in terms of money, this lack of adequate income did not help the professor's social standing. It is no wonder that scientists and other academic persons played no such roles in government or public affairs, as did their European colleagues.

Gibbs, for personal reasons, was content in this situation. He had his own income and cared little about public recognition. But not many scientists could subsidize their own research; and even those who could do this, were discouraged by public attitudes from devoting themselves to "useless" studies. Dr. Samuel Jackson, of the University of Pennsylvania, pointed out in 1840 that even a wealthy physician must cultivate a fashionable practice, and thereby neglect research, if he wished to secure either public or professional recognition.[16] And the best known physical scientists were those who, like Benjamin Silliman of Yale, gave a large part of their time to teaching, geologic surveys, and popular lecturing.[17]

The blighting effect of utilitarianism was evident in the diversion of men who showed promise in basic research into applied activities. Silliman may have illustrated this, though one cannot be certain in individual cases. European professors were puzzled by American students who, after beginning well abroad, lapsed into mediocrity upon returning home. And one recalls cases in which Americans, inspired by European science, actually began to make basic contributions, but never went on to a fulfillment of the potentialities so revealed. Thus

[16] *Address to the Medical Graduates of the University of Pennsylvania,* T. K. Collins, Philadelphia, 1840, p. 15.
[17] John F. Fulton and E. H. Thomson, *Benjamin Silliman,* Henry Schuman, New York, 1947, *passim.*

Samuel Gross did original work in pathologic anatomy and published in 1839 the first real text on that subject in any language; but he became so involved in teaching and surgical practice that the time he could give to autopsies became quite inadequate.[18] Hence his ultimate contribution to the field was less than that of his great European contemporaries.

The same withering influence was to be observed in the failure to recognize such basic work as Americans did accomplish, despite all handicaps. Such exceptional men as Gibbs, or the physiologist William Beaumont, were more appreciated in Europe than in their own country. Joseph Henry, who pursued basic work in electro-magnetics which paralleled that of Faraday, was not as well known in America as was Samuel Morse, although the latter simply applied Henry's discoveries to the making of a commercially successful telegraph.[19]

Was the extreme emphasis upon utility an old or new note in American science? Among eighteenth century scientists, especially in the American Philosophical Society, the conscious direction of research toward human welfare had been demanded in the traditional Baconian manner. William Smith, provost of the University of Pennsylvania, declared in 1790 that: "The man who will . . . point out a new and profitable article of agriculture and commerce, will deserve more from his fellow citizens and from heaven, than all the Latin and Greek scholars, or all the teachers of technical learning, that ever existed, in any age or country." [20] And the motivation of many of the colonial planters and merchants, who pursued science as an avocation, was plainly a utilitarian

[18] Edgar Goldschmid, "Contributions des Etats-Unis à l'Anatomie pathologique au début du xixᵉ siècle," *Archives internationales d'Histoire des Sciences*, 1948, n° 3, pp. 479 ff.

[19] Bernard Jaffe, *Men of Science in America,* Simon and Schuster, New York, 1944, pp. 193 ff.

[20] J. Bell Whitfield, "The Scientific Environment of Philadelphia, 1775–1790," *Proceedings,* American Philosophical Society (Philadelphia), vol. 92, n°1, 1948, pp. 10, 11.

one. Against this background, American attitudes during the
nineteenth century seemed to represent a persistence of those
of the earlier period.

A closer analysis, however, reveals that in the later age
subtle changes occurred in the nature of science and also in
the composition of society. In the first place, and despite
formal statements to the contrary, some of the best work of the
older leaders had been of a basic sort, or had been—in any
case—motivated by pure intellectual curiosity. This was true,
for example, of the ablest Philadelphians—of Bartram, Rittenhouse, Benjamin Rush and Franklin.[21] Since science had then
been relatively non-technical and could be cultivated by self-
trained men, there was nothing to prevent gifted persons from
pursuing it in their spare time. If their interests were abstract
or "impractical," that was their own concern as amateurs and
who was to say them nay? Either basic or applied studies could
be made, under these circumstances, as their authors desired.

Between 1800 and 1850, however, science rapidly became
relatively complex and technical. This trend required more
formal training, more specializing, and more professionalization.[22] And when men made their living as scientists, they
could not pursue their own curiosity with the same freedom as
could amateurs. If the surrounding society would support pure
research—as in the German universities—well and good. But
if society disdained this, as in the United States, it was apt to

[21] Rush attempted to solve what he believed were the basic problems in
pathology, though his approach now seems speculative; see Shryock,
"Benjamin Rush from the Perspective of the Twentieth Century,"
Transactions, College of Physicians of Philadelphia, 4 series, vol. 14, n° 3,
Déc. 1946, pp. 114 ff. On Franklin's basic research, see Cohen, *op. cit.*

[22] J. D. Bernal, *The Social Function of Science,* Macmillan, New York,
1939, pp. 28, 29, notes professionalization, and adds that it was
accompanied by the withdrawal of scientists from "the direction of State
and of industry." Perhaps this was because government and business were
also becoming more complex.

be neglected. Thus changes in the nature of science itself accounted in part for the American situation under discussion.

In the second place, American society underwent a transformation, between 1780 and 1830, from a relatively aristocratic to a relatively democratic one. Prior to the latter year, there had been some "patrician" support of science as well as of art —a persistence of the European type of patronage.[23] Although the merchants and planters of 1750 or 1800 possessed a middle-class background, they aspired to gentility and represented in a sense the American aristocracy. Even those individuals in this class who pursued science themselves were really patrons, since they supported the work from income derived from other sources.

This situation changed when, after about 1830, equalitarianism ("Jacksonian democracy") permeated American society. There was a "decline of aristocracy" in science as well as in politics. Wealthy gentlemen who devoted themselves to pure research became rare, and individuals who did so—for example, the psychologist Dr. James Rush—were apt to be viewed as eccentric.

Tocqueville recognized the connection between equalitarianism and the neglect of basic science during the 1830's. By that time, American apologists were proclaiming that applied science was the peculiar glory of a democracy, since only in such a society would science be put to work for the benefit of the masses.[24] But it is doubtful if the emphasis upon utility was to be ascribed directly to "the multitude" or to the "working classes" to which Tocqueville referred. There is every evidence that businessmen became a more dominant class between 1830 and 1900 than they had been before that time. Equalitarianism influenced them, not by weakening

---

[23] Curti, *op. cit.*, pp. 213 ff.
[24] *Ibid.*, pp. 333 ff.

their power, but by making this more economic than social in nature. Technology made possible new and greater fortunes, at the same time that equalitarianism undermined certain social ideals which had tempered the older quest for wealth.

In other words, such categories as "middle class" or even "business men" are too inclusive for the present purpose. The textile manufacturers of 1850 or the railroad magnates of 1875 apparently sought wealth as a means to power, and accumulated more than could be used for personal comfort or even for social display. Their neglect of the genteel tradition and its cultural implications probably resulted from a number of circumstances. They were *nouveau riche,* in a day when equalitarianism had robbed gentility of much of its older prestige. Moreover, they were business men at a time when business—like science—was becoming more complex and technical. The very scale and tempo of industrial expansion, especially after 1850, was such as to absorb all a man's time and interest. We do not yet have adequate studies of the thought of this class—of their folklore, ideals, rationalizations and so on. But they seem to have been more ruthless than were the older merchants or planters in demanding efficiency and profits.[25]

Far from challenging this sense of values, the masses made it their own. Could not even the common man "get ahead" in the American environment by emulating the millionaires? Thus the ideals of our business leaders became the ideals of the great majority of the people, though only a few were themselves endowed with the talent for leadership." [26] Under these circumstances, "radical" movements like Marxian socialism made small appeal; hence the masses received no such

[25] Thomas E. Cochran and William Miller, *The Age of Enterprise: A Social History of Industrial America,* Macmillan, New York, 1942, pp. 67 ff.
[26] *Ibid.,* p. 153.

indoctrination in the values of science as might have come from that source. They either accepted unconsciously the business man's evaluations, or remained indifferent to the whole matter.

Industrial leaders, on the other hand, were in a position to support basic science if they had so desired. Without waiting for mass enlightenment or possible government aid, they could have provided philanthropic endowments or direct subsidies for corporation research. But of all intellectual or cultural activities, theoretical science was the least likely to appeal to them. The most ruthless magnate might enjoy literature of some sort and appreciate the ornamental quality of the fine arts, but why should he encourage the "idle curiosity" of research men? Such curiosity, to him, was neither interesting nor ornamental. There was nothing in his own experience to suggest that out of basic science would come—ultimately— applications and profits. And although this probability already had been demonstrated in the past, the self-made industrialist was not usually familiar with so "impractical" a subject as the history of science.

Even if they had known the ultimate value of theoretical science for technology, it is doubtful if "big business men" would have supported the former as long as the connection seemed remote. Living in a highly competitive, "get-rich-quick" environment, they were interested in immediate rather than in ultimate results. There was an analogy here with the common tendency of most Americans, farmers as well as manufacturers, to exploit the resources of the moment without regard to the long-run consequences.

It is true that merchants and manufacturers were sometimes defended against those who condemned their materialism, and that this defense included the claim that their activities encouraged science. The view here advanced by conservative Americans was, strangely enough, similar to that emphasized by many later Marxists; that is, that the greater part of science had in the past grown out of response to economic needs.[27] But even in such analyses, it was clear that Americans conceived of science primarily in terms of its applications, and were hardly conscious of theoretical science as such.[28]

The proof of the role of business men in the American neglect of basic research, prior to about 1900, is to be observed in their support of this same process after that time. The rather sudden emergence of basic science in the United States can be largely ascribed to the support of business leaders —support which was provided only after science had reached a point where its implications for technology became more apparent. There was, between 1900 and 1940, a gradual increase in popular appreciation of the relations between basic and applied research, and a consequent growth of government aid for both procedures. But this was preceded by more immediate aid extended to basic science by private wealth. Indeed, both popular interest and government subsidies may be interpreted as a response to the earlier research achievements of the universities, foundations, and corporations which were financed so largely in this recent era by business leaders.[29]

In conclusion, we may revert for a moment—for comparative purposes—to one other phenomenon for which Tocqueville's analysis failed to account. This was the successful cultivation of American literature during the nineteenth century, in contrast to the relative neglect of basic science. The French observer was correct in believing that equalitarianism would influence literature, but was misled in the view

[27] *Cf.* Bernal, *op. cit.,* pp. 20 ff.; and J. Pelseneer, "Les Influences dans l'Histoire des Sciences," *Archives Internationales d'Histoire des Sciences,* n° 3 (1948), p. 352 (Nouvelle Série d *Archeion,* tome XXVII).

[28] See, e.g., "The American Merchant," *The Knickerbocker or New-York Monthly Magazine,* vol. 14 (1839), pp. 10 ff., 118.

[29] Shryock, *American Medical Research,* pp. 53 ff., 90 ff.

that the quality of this art would decline under the leveling impact of democracy. There were, of course, critics who lamented the influence of commercialism and of vulgar taste upon the arts; and there was certainly much that was banal in the popular literary output. But what happened in the long run was that superior literature—as it has been judged abroad, as well as in the United States—was diverted and modified, rather than inhibited by mass tastes and the dominance of business ideals.

As soon as literary forms of high quality could be adapted to the tastes of a relatively large public, there was an actual advantage to authors in the widespread literacy of a democracy. Earlier than in any other country, the United States produced a literature written by the middle classes and aimed at the masses. Outstanding authors, from Bryant to Mark Twain, consciously cultivated forms which were—to use Poe's phrase—"more appreciable by the mass of mankind." [30] There was no analogy to this situation in basic science, since the latter was not susceptible to democratic adaptations. "Popular science" was not, and cannot be, basic science, whereas literature may be simultaneously popular and of high quality.

In summing up this analysis, one observes that the very middle class which did much for science during the early modern centuries, neglected in the United States to aid fundamental studies throughout most of the nineteenth century. It is not surprising, in view of all the circumstances noted, that "pure" science (motivated by pure curiosity) made little headway. But it is rather striking that so little basic research grew out of extensive applied activities. It seems clear, therefore, that economic interests and technology will not of themselves lead automatically into basic investigations. Other variables influence the outcome.

[30] Clarence Gohdes, *American Literature in Nineteenth-Century England,* Columbia University Press, New York, 1944, pp. 11, 12.

The industry of the nineteenth century (including American) needed basic research as well as technology. Indeed, this need was probably greater than that of any preceding economic order. Yet the industrialists were more responsible than any other class, at least in the United States, for all the indifference which has been described. This apparent paradox cannot be fully explained by reference to the laissez faire principles upheld in Britain and America during this period. These principles were opposed to government planning and even to government aid for science, but would not in themselves have discouraged private support.[31] In the United States, moreover, the laissez faire philosophy was hardly established until after mid-century, and it will be noted that it was never sufficiently strong to prevent the considerable government assistance to applied science which has been mentioned.

A more complete explanation of American neglect may be found in the analysis of simultaneous changes in the nature of science and in the composition of society, each of which interacted on the other in a complex manner. A more technical and specialized science, on the one hand, and a more equalitarian and industrialized society on the other, each played a part in producing the end results.

It seems clear that industrial society failed—to a large extent in Britain, but even more completely in the United States—to support basic science from any motive whatsoever. Where more or less aristocratic institutions survived, however, there was maintained, or evolved, a tradition of "pure" science which resulted in much basic research. (Whether, in certain countries, more such research also grew out of technology than was the case in the United States, is a question which cannot be considered here.)

[31] *Cf.* Bernal, *op. cit.,* pp. 27, 28.

Aristocratic support was never very strong in the United States and largely disappeared there after 1830. It was more persistent in England, but flourished most in the German and other Continental universities. The latter system, with its support of "pure" science, doubtless suffered from a lack of planning and coordination, and perhaps also involved some studies which led nowhere in terms of ultimate social values. But it had the merit of assuring complete freedom to individual scientists; and this permitted the greatest among them to open up hitherto unknown and therefore unpredictable areas which subsequently proved of the greatest utility.

In a word, aristocratic support enabled basic science to advance to a technical point at which its value for industry became apparent even to the industrialists. At present, in the United States, leading industrialists and the scientists associated with them are fully aware of the significance of fundamental studies. More than this, some of these leaders are convinced that those studies which are motivated by pure curiosity often prove of the greatest utility—even if measured in crass financial terms.[32] But the chief emphasis upon "pure" science has developed since about 1890 in the research institutes and in the universities. It is probably true that in both government and industrial science, the major American emphasis continues to relate to applied studies, or to such types of basic investigation as seem to promise most for utility in the near future.

[32] For an illustration of this, see the remarks of Irving Langmuir in the *Dedication* volume, Lilly Research Laboratories, Eli Lilly and Co., Indianapolis, 1934, pp. 7 ff.

IV

A Medical Perspective
on the Civil War *

Among the various themes pertinent to Civil War history, medicine seems least apt to lend itself to centennial celebrations. Do we really wish to recall, a century later, the incredible suffering which occurred on battlefields and in hospitals during that conflict? One would judge, from much recent writing on the War itself, that there is no such desire. Yet, if medical aspects are omitted, the story is not only incomplete but is unrealistic as a total picture. It can provide analyses of military strategy or may portray the day to day life of troops in the field. But often it becomes a dramatic narrative which, though containing vivid accounts of battle scenes, fails to make real the tragedy inherent in the entire experience.

What actually happened was that a struggle which began almost light-heartedly at Bull Run soon became one of the bloodiest wars of all time. A number of circumstances converged to make it so. First, this was a people's war and large numbers of troops were involved—perhaps three million all told. Second, although morale was not always high, armies sought out opponents with much determination. Third, in combat, most wounds were caused by musket or rifle fire, and the leaden bullets then employed did more damage than do

* Reprinted from the *American Quarterly*, XIV (Summer, 1962)—by permission.

modern, steel counterparts. Fourth, surgical practice was such that nearly all penetrating wounds were fatal except those of the extremities, and even the latter had a high mortality rate.

Most appalling, however, was the fact that many wounded who might have been saved were abandoned on battlefields. No adequate ambulance services and field hospitals were available as late as 1862. At Second Bull Run, for example, the Union army was supposed to have 170 ambulances, but actually went into battle with 45—most of which broke down. Several days after the battle, in consequence, 3,000 wounded still lay where they had fallen. In this situation, many men bled to death or died from exposure and were then reported as "killed in action." Worse still, in certain instances—as at Chancellorsville in '63 and again at the Wilderness in '64— hundreds of the wounded actually burned to death when shells set the woods on fire.

After ambulance facilities were provided, field hospitals were sometimes overwhelmed by major-battle casualties. At Gettysburg, for example, the Union medical corps was well equipped with 1,000 ambulances, 650 officers, and about 3,000 drivers and stretchermen. But within three days, 21,000 wounded were brought in just when most of the medical officers were moving on with the army. Each remaining surgeon was thus left with an average of 900 cases on his hands.[1] Haste and neglect were unavoidable under such circumstances.

Those among the wounded who *were* properly tended in field and base hospitals had still to run the risks of surgery. As is well known, anesthetics were usually available, but there

[1] George W. Adams, *Doctors in Blue* (New York: Henry Schuman, 1952), pp. 91 f. See also T. M. Hunter, "Medical Service for the Yankee Soldier" (thesis, University of Maryland, 1952), *passim*. Both of these studies are thorough and indicate the wide ranges of sources relating to the present subject.

was no notion of aseptic procedures. Looking back in 1918, the Philadelphia surgeon W. W. Keen recalled that: [2]

> We operated in old blood-stained and often pus-stained coats . . . with undisinfected hands. . . . We used undisinfected instruments . . . and marine sponges which had been used in prior pus cases and only washed in tap water.

No wonder that nearly all wounds became infected and that there was still some talk of "laudable pus" in the medieval manner. In the case of chest or abdominal wounds, surgeons probed with their fingers, prescribed morphine and tried to stop external bleeding. Otherwise, there was little they could do. The victims usually died within three days from hemorrhage and/or infection. The average Union mortality from gunshot wounds of the chest was 62 per cent of cases; and from such wounds of the abdomen, no less than 87 per cent.[3] By way of contrast, only about 3 per cent of all American wounded failed to survive in World War II.[4]

Chances were better but not too good with injuries of the extremities, for joints could be removed or limbs amputated. It is difficult to find mortality rates for amputations, but they were certainly high by modern standards. Here again, it was usually the ensuing infection which caused death—the so-called "surgical fevers" which included tetanus, erysipelas, hospital-gangrene and pyemia ("blood poisoning").

The infectious nature of wound gangrene was recognized and cases were isolated in hospitals when feasible. Efforts were also made to disinfect wounds, as when bromine was used

[2] W. W. Keen, "Military Surgery in 1861 and in 1918," *Annals American Academy of Political and Social Science*, LXXX (1918), 11 ff.

[3] Adams, *Doctors in Blue*, p. 135.

[4] R. H. Shryock, *American Medical Research: Past and Present* (New York: Commonwealth Fund, 1947), p. 294.

with some success against this same disease. Among the chemicals so employed was carbolic acid, the very agent which Lister used soon thereafter in the first demonstrations of antiseptic surgery. This being the case, why did not the Civil War surgeons anticipate Lister? Since they thought that carbolic would clean out infected wounds, why did they not use it to sterilize fresh wounds and instruments in the first place?

The difference on which the outcomes turned was largely a theoretical one. Lister, impressed by Pasteur's view of bacterial origins of infection, assumed that the surgeon's hand or instrument was introducing pathogenic organisms. Ergo, if wounds were sprayed at the start with carbolic acid, infection could be avoided. But American surgeons of the 1860's were either unfamiliar with bacteriology or did not take it seriously. They were "practical men" with more wound experience than was possessed by any surgeons elsewhere, yet this did not prevent them from adhering to another old theory; namely, that infections were caused by "noxious miasms" arising from filth and carried through the air.

It followed that the way to prevent wound infection was to avoid these miasms. And this could be done by seeking ordinary cleanliness in hospitals—by carrying over into these institutions the sanitary controls already demanded in public hygiene. Surgeons, it was assumed, had nothing to do with introducing infectious poisons: the latter were just literally "in the air." But once infection appeared in a wound, the surgeon could then attempt to *dis*infect it by applying chemicals. All this was logical enough but we can now see that it was these practical men who were ultimately impractical. Their chemotherapy for already-infected wounds often came too late.

Cumulative experience enabled surgeons to improve certain techniques, as in handling the great arteries. Occasionally a new and useful procedure emerged, only to be forgotten after the War and perhaps reintroduced many years later.[5] A striking illustration of this resulted from pure chance. Several Southern doctors, lacking supplies for keeping maggots out of wounds, found that these visitors actually cleaned out dead tissue and prevented infection.[6] This fact had been stumbled upon during the Napoleonic Wars, was rediscovered in the '60's as noted, then was overlooked again and finally discovered for the third time—much to everyone's amazement—during World War I. Empirical findings of this sort, based simply on trial and error, were usually known only to those immediately involved and were then easily forgotten. In the case mentioned, most surgeons continued conscientiously to remove maggots and thus assured infection. In other words, incidental technical advances did little to check mortality resulting from wounds.

Statistical data on military losses vary widely, but it has been stated that as many as 110,000 Northern soldiers and 94,000 Southerners succumbed to battle injuries. One may roughly estimate from these data that from 6 to 10 per cent of Union troops and from 10 to 15 per cent of the Confederate troops died from wounds. The exact ratios depend on what estimates are accepted for the total number of troops involved.

High as were the casualties, it is well known that losses from disease were higher. While 110,000 Union soldiers perished from wounds, some 250,000 died from disease: the corresponding figures for Confederates were probably about 94,000 and 164,000. The average soldier, as a matter of fact, was ill between two and three times each year, and the annual

[5] Such a lost technique is described in L. L. Schwartz, "James Bolton," *American Journal of Surgery*, n.s., LXI (December, 1944), 409.

[6] H. H. Cunningham, *Doctors in Grey* (Baton Rouge: Louisiana State University Press, 1958), p. 234.

mortality from sickness was more than 5 per cent. Compared with male civilians of military age, servicemen were five times as likely to become ill and experienced a mortality which was five times as high as that of those who remained at home.[7]

Strangely enough, from the present viewpoint, army leaders thought their record very creditable—even when as many as 10 per cent of all troops were ill at one time. Actually, the record *was* creditable in comparison with preceding wars: it is only in contrast with later conflicts that the medical experience of 1861–65 seems so startling. Thus, while the annual disease mortality rate was then about 53 per thousand soldiers, this ratio fell to 16 per thousand during the Spanish War, and to about 12 per thousand during World War I.[8] In other words, the disease death rate for troops during the Civil War was more than four times as great as that experienced in 1917–18.

The explanation of this relatively high mortality was not as simple as one might think. In the first place, the limitations of wound surgery were those of medicine in general. The War came just too soon to witness certain major advances in hygiene and surgery. If it could have been postponed for two decades, many deaths would have been avoided.

Even at that, the knowledge already available in 1861 would have made possible much lower mortality rates if it had only been applied effectively. The utter lack of preparation and subsequent inefficiency in the medical services must bear much of the blame for unnecessary illness. This inefficiency was not the fault of any one group. Sharing in responsibility were the original medical officers, indifferent generals and politicians, a mediocre profession, and rural regiments hitherto

[7] See T. G. Livermore, *Numbers and Losses in the Civil War: 1861–1865* (New York: Houghton Mifflin Co., 1901), pp. 5–8.

[8] Adams, *Doctors in Blue*, pp. 222–24.

unexposed to infections and unfamiliar with the rudiments of hygiene. Over against such villains of the piece must be placed the many heroic figures. Among the latter were certain generals, such as McClellan, who supported reform in the medical services; a growing number of conscientious Army surgeons; and a host of civilian volunteers who called for better medical care and meantime ministered directly to those in need.

The chief diseases among troops were caused directly or indirectly by unhealthy environments and bad habits. In the early War years, sanitation in hastily constructed camps was crude at best. Both food and water supplies were infected, and typhoid, dysentery, and diarrhea became the most common and most fatal of camp afflictions. White, Union troops had an average annual rate of 711 cases and 15 deaths from these diseases for every thousand men. The gastro-enteritis problem was complicated by the standard ration of beans, salt beef and army biscuits, as well as by the men's habit of frying everything as long as they did their own cooking. Gastronomically, one can hardly imagine a worse regimen, and it is no wonder that there was some scurvy (13 cases annually per 1,000) as well as endless "dyspepsia."

The second most common type of illness was malaria, which involved an average annual rate of 522 cases per 1,000 Union troops but only 3 deaths. More fatal were the respiratory infections, resulting from exposure in the field and overcrowding in tents or barracks. Tuberculosis was serious, though its mortality was not recorded. What was termed "inflammation of the lungs" presumably included the pneumonias and was responsible among Union troops for an average of 6 deaths per 1,000 men each year. Rheumatism was common and there was an unknown amount of alcoholism and of mental illness. Measles and mumps were annoying but not fatal, and the same was thought to be true of venereal diseases.[9]

Although a higher proportion of officers than of enlisted men were killed in battle, the latter suffered a disease mortality rate about twice as high as that for officers. Rural troops, until adjusted to crowded camp life, endured more illness than did urban soldiers; which may explain why Western volunteers had a sick rate in 1861 more than twice as high as that for Easterners. Illness was always more common and more fatal among Negro than with white troops: the lung infections which killed 6 white men per thousand annually, resulted in no less than 28 deaths among a corresponding number of Negroes. More significant was the relatively high mortality from disease among Confederate as compared with Union soldiers, especially from respiratory infections. During the first eighteen months of the War "half again as many Confederates died of diarrhea and dysentery, while more than *five times* as many died of pulmonary diseases." [10]

It is hard to believe that there was so great a contrast between Union and Confederate mortality; but, if true, the excessive Southern losses may be hypothetically explained by unfamiliarity with northern winters and by the relative scarcity of food, clothing, and drugs during the latter part of the War. On both sides, of course, resistance to infections was lowered by exposure or malnutrition. These and other adverse circumstances also lessened a man's chances in undergoing surgery.

In treating disease in the 1860's, medical men were at some

[9] Morbidity and mortality data are given in the *Medical and Surgical History of the War of the Rebellion;* e.g., Pt. II, Vol. I (Washington, D.C.: Government Printing Office, 1879), pp. 1–40. See also the reports issued by the U.S. Sanitary Commission; e.g., Document No. 71 (New York: U.S. Sanitary Commission, 1863).

[10] Adams, *Doctors in Blue,* p. 14.

disadvantage in comparison with both their predecessors of 1760 and their successors of 1960. They obviously lacked many present aids—the antibiotics, for example, or the resources of aseptic surgery. They did possess certain helpful drugs unknown during the Revolution, notably quinine against malaria and chloroform as an anesthetic. But, just because medical science had become more critical after 1820, Civil War surgeons had little of that confidence in traditional remedies which had heartened practitioners in earlier years.

Actually, there was more skepticism about the value of drugs during the later nineteenth century than in any other period before or since. Medical leaders had learned to distrust the old, therapeutic standbys of bleeding and purging but had as yet found few new remedies in their place. Bleeding was already frowned upon during the 1850's; and although some older doctors continued it into the '70's, it was little employed during the Civil War. If a man lost blood on the field, he was not subjected—as in Revolutionary days—to further bleeding in the hospital. And although emetics and laxatives, along with morphine and whiskey, were routine remedies, the chief medical officers shared a growing distrust of extreme vomiting and purging. This distrust found expression in an order issued by Union Surgeon General Hammond in 1863, banning the use of the mercurials, tartar emetic and calomel. Some military surgeons resisted this order, which definitely reduced their "armamentarium." But the episode pointed in the direction which medical practice would follow thereafter.

A less fortunate aspect of medical thought at mid-century was its emphasis upon specific diseases rather than—as in earlier days—on the general state of the patient's "system." This emphasis upon specificity pointed toward the identification of particular illnesses, and how to discover causes or cures until the diseases themselves were first known? But, meantime, inquiring physicians became more interested in diseases, or in injuries as such, than in the patients who harbored them. Instead of being concerned about the total condition of John Smith in ward B, they were intrigued by the "strange case" of typhoid or by the "extraordinary wounds" found in this same location. Modern medicine, in contrast, has returned to older concern about complete physiologic reactions to disease or injury. Thus, reports on World War II wounds often relate to kidney involvement in resulting "shock," whereas those of the Civil War were limited to the immediate, structural damage involved.

The emphasis of the 1860's on specificity not only over-looked generalized pathology but also gave little heed to the patient's state of mind. Laymen sensed this situation at times, as when Louisa Alcott remarked of a surgeon in Washington that he: [11]

> had acquired a somewhat trying habit of regarding a man and his wound [or illness] as separate institutions, and seemed rather annoyed that the former should express any opinion on the latter, or claim any right in it, while under his care,

Speaking elsewhere of the same surgeon, she added that: [12]

> The more intricate the wound, the better he liked it. A poor private, with both legs off, and shot through the lungs, possessed more attractions for him than a dozen generals slightly scratched in some "masterly retreat."

The tendency to focus on diseases rather than on patients reflected the best hospital standards of the day. Back in the homes whence enlisted men had come, family doctors probably still viewed their patients as persons and not simply as "cases" of this or that; but in hospitals—including the military

[11] Louisa M. Alcott, *Hospital Sketches* (Cambridge, Harvard University Press, 1960—1st ed., 1863), p. 87.
[12] Alcott, *Hospital Sketches*, p. 37.

—such over-all concern was often lost. It would have been lessened in any case, within army circles, by the tendency to give routine care to masses of sick or injured soldiers. One suspects that most medical officers, practicing a form of "State medicine," had neither time nor inclination to cultivate solicitude or even bedside manners.

Both scientific attitudes and military circumstances thus set limits to the effectiveness of the medical care provided. But, within these limits, what was the general quality of those who served on both sides as medical officers? At the start, most of these men had had little surgical experience, since specialization in surgery was still unknown in this country. It also must be remembered that the effort to train first-class practitioners (real physicians) had not yet had much success in America in 1860; indeed, would not fully succeed until the present century. Many medical schools were mediocre or worse, even by the standards of the time; and much the same thing can be said of most of their graduates. There had been frequent criticism of "regular" practitioners before 1860, as ignoramuses who killed their patients with the lancet and calomel; and such distrust, carrying over into the War years, apparently influenced attitudes in both the Army and in Congress.

On the other hand, a few first-rate physicians—some of them professors from the better schools—joined the medical departments or served as contract surgeons in base hospitals. Men of this stamp had taken postdoctoral work in Paris during the 1830's and '40's, and by the '50's were turning to Vienna for such training. A few of them had developed research interests while abroad. But the War temporarily checked migration to the Austrian center, and its demands on medical personnel left little time for investigations in pathology or physiology. The chief exceptions to this rule grew out of clinical studies based directly on hospital observations, as in the work done by W. W. Keen on nerve injuries.

Technical improvements in surgery also grew directly out of empirical experience. Although these achievements, as noted, had little effect on mortality rates, they did gain recognition abroad for American surgery. Even before 1860 Europeans had been impressed by American prowess in dental and in gynecologic operations. And since Civil War experience promoted military surgery in general, there was much foreign acclaim of "manipulative skills" in this country.

After the War, American surgical instruments were highly praised at an 1868 exposition in Paris. Even more impressive was the subsequent publication, by the U.S. Army Medical Department, of the ponderous *Medical and Surgical History of the War of the Rebellion* (1870–88), wherein masses of pathologic data were made available. The German pathologist, Virchow, said of these collections that: [13]

> Whoever . . . reads the extensive publications of the American medical staff will be constantly astonished at the wealth of experience therein found. The greatest exactness in detail, careful statistics, . . . and a scholarly statement . . . are here united, to preserve and transmit . . . the knowledge purchased at so vast an expense.

Probably the highest foreign praise accorded Civil War doctors was that expressed by the Swiss physician Edwin Klebs. Writing in the '80's, Klebs declared that: [14]

> . . . the greatest and most admirable success has been attained by the North Americans in military medical work. The history of the war of the secession has to show a display of medical and scientific activities that leave anything that ever since has been achieved in Europe way in the background. . . .

[13] Quoted in Francis R. Packard, *History of Medicine in the United States,* I (New York: Paul B. Hoeber, 1931), 650.

[14] Edwin Klebs, in the *Deutsche Medicinischen Wochenschrift* for 1881–83, quoted in T. N. Bonner, "American Doctors and German Universities: 1870–1914" (MS.), pp. 13 f.

Perhaps Klebs was a bit too appreciative. At any rate, granting that medical records were well preserved and granting also that surgeons acquired manipulative skill, it remains true that little that was basically new emerged from the War experience. This has usually been the case with war medicine. American physicians who had done little research before 1861 were still less inclined to pursue it under military pressures. As a matter of fact, they did not even keep up with new methods or instruments introduced in Europe from one to three decades earlier. Such simple, diagnostic procedures as the use of clinical thermometers and of stethoscopes were rarely employed in the military services.

If much of the medical story of the Civil War seems depressing today, it did at least have its brighter side. There is no better way of presenting this than to forget the armed forces for the moment and to recall rather the civilian welfare organizations. The tradition of voluntary help in emergencies had already been established before 1861, as in the work of the so-called Howard associations during epidemics. But the Civil War called for such aid on a vastly increased scale. Women's relief agencies, in the form of local hospital societies or even of such state-wide bodies as the Georgia Relief and Hospital Association, were formed in the Confederacy.[15] But only in the Union, where states' rights were not taken so seriously, did such efforts result in the founding of regional or national organizations—notably of the Christian Commission, the Western Sanitary Commission, and the United States Sanitary Commission. Of these, the last-named was most significant.

Seeking at first just to be helpful, women's relief societies were formed in Boston and in New York City in 1861. These and other groups coalesced into the U.S. Sanitary Commis-

---

[15] Cunningham, *Doctors in Grey*, p. 22.

sion, acquired able directors and officers, and were officially recognized in Washington. But their representatives were appalled by the chaos they found there, and particularly by the hopeless inefficiency of the Army medical corps. Protesting against resulting suffering among the troops, they were rebuffed by the Secretary of War as meddlers and termed by Lincoln a mere "fifth wheel" for the military agencies. That did it! From this time on, the Commission—directed by the able Frederick Law Olmsted—investigated, reported, and successfully pressured the services into the reform of medical care both in the field and in hospitals. Their inspiration came from the sanitary ideal of the era: the conviction that pure water, good food, fresh air, and general cleanliness would prevent nearly all human ills.

This is not the place to recall the endless negotiations of the Commission with cabinet members, field commanders, medical officers, and congressmen.[16] But out of its efforts, and those of enlightened Army personnel, came improved camp sanitation, the use of ambulances, the combination of regimental into divisional field hospitals, the building of pavilion-plan base hospitals, and the encouragement of nursing by women.

The greater part of so-called nursing in military hospitals was done by convalescent soldiers, who lacked training, aptitude, and strength for the work. But Florence Nightingale's achievements in the Crimea had aroused interest in the possible services of women. Hence the Union War Department commissioned Dorothea Dix as the first Superintendent of Army Nurses; that is, of women in this program. Those who volunteered received little training but had to meet certain requirements, such as being strong, middle-aged and of plain appearance. (Miss Dix would have no nonsense

[16] The latest and most complete study of the Commission is that of William Q. Maxwell, *Lincoln's Fifth Wheel* (New York: Longmans, Green & Co., 1956).

in her outfit.) Most of these women made up in idealism what they lacked in other respects and so were able to do much for the morale of their patients. How important this could be, from a medical as well as from a humane viewpoint, was probably not as fully realized in the 1860's as it has been in recent decades.

The reminiscences of the volunteer nurses provide vivid pictures of suffering observed within base hospitals. (After all, such mortality statistics as have been noted here are abstractions: they provide basic data but are far removed from human experience.) Further lines from Alcott's *Sketches,* for example, will make the hospital picture more real than will all the figures in the world. Perhaps the following account of a boy's sudden death will serve our purpose.

Observing that a patient had not eaten his meal, Miss Alcott offered him coffee, whereupon he startled her by saying simply: "Thank you, ma'am; I don't think I'll ever eat again, for I'm shot in the stomach. But I'd like a drink of water, if you aint too busy:" [17]

> I rushed away [continues Miss Alcott] but the water pails were gone to be refilled, and it was some time before they reappeared. I did not forget my patient patient, meanwhile, and, with the first mugfull, hurried back to him. He seemed asleep; but something in the tired white face caused me to listen at his lips for a breath. None came . . . and then I knew that, while he waited, a better nurse than I had . . . healed him with a touch . . . half an hour later, the bed was empty. It seemed a poor requital for all he had . . . suffered—that hospital bed, lonely even in a crowd; for there was no familiar face . . . no friendly voice to say, Good-bye; no hand to lead him gently down into the Valley

---

[17] Alcott, *Hospital Sketches,* pp. 36 f. General accounts of women as nurses are given in M. B. Greenbie, *Lincoln's Daughters of Mercy* (New York: G. P. Putnam's Sons, 1944). On Miss Dix, see Helen E. Marshall, *Dorothea Lynde Dix: A Forgotten Samaritan* (Chapel Hill: University of North Carolina Press, 1936).

of the Shadow. . . . For a moment I felt bitterly indignant
at this seeming carelessness of the value of life . . . then
consoled myself with the thought that, when the great
muster roll was called, these nameless men might be
promoted above many whose tall monuments record the
barren honors they have won.

Present readers may think this only Victorian sentimentality, and one must admit that modern writers might handle
the same theme somewhat differently. Yet I sense in these
lines, written by a New England girl almost one hundred
years ago, a genuine and moving experience. By implication,
moreover, the statement raises one of the eternal questions
about war which may be posed here again in summing up the
whole matter. Putting aside any thought of pacifism in
principle, how can we balance suffering over against achievements in order to decide whether this particular conflict was
really worth its cost? Did the aftermath fully compensate for
the loss of some 600,000 young lives—to say nothing of
further anguish among those who survived?

Obviously, such matters cannot be reduced to quantitative
terms. There is no magic arithmetic which can multiply the
value of one life by 600,000 and come up with a meaningful
total. And if there were, who could determine for comparison
the tangible merit of one Union or the real value of emancipation—even if we assume that these goals could have been
attained only by combat? Although such questions cannot be
answered with finality, they are not necessarily devoid of
meaning. In the fullness of time, they may have some bearing
on ultimate conclusions.

We do not often ponder the medical record of the Civil
War.[18] Other sources recall other evil consequences but it is

---

[18] A striking exception to this, published since the preparation of the
present paper, is Allan Nevins' article "The Glorious and the Terrible," in
the *Saturday Review*, XLIV, No. 35 (Sept. 2, 1961), 9 ff.; which
emphasizes suffering in the Civil War. Nevins also points out other

this record which best suggests the full measure of human costs. One may emphasize the point by raising a simple question: What part of the country still recalls "the War" most persistently? Obviously, the South. Why? Because, we are told, that section lost more and suffered more. But did it? Well yes, in humiliation or bitterness, and—as Professor Nichols has made clear—in power as well as in property. *But not in lives.* If the usual estimates may be depended on, almost 100,000 more Northern men than Southern died in this holocaust.[19]

Yet for all our protestations about the sanctity of life, these vital losses present that aspect of war which is most soon forgotten. Such an outcome may be ascribed in part to the common habit of suppressing unhappy memories, but more than this has been involved. Consider, for example, Professor Woodward's observation that Southerners, in recalling defeat and ruin in 1865, are the only Americans who have any memory of national frustration.[20] It follows, by implication, that the death of thousands of fathers and sons in the North aroused no lasting feeling of this nature. Where victory was followed by prosperity, there was hardly even a surviving awareness of national tragedy.

These rather acrid thoughts are consistent with one's personal impressions. Over the years, I have known only one

---

unhappy results which, though not pertinent here, have to be weighed in any final judgment on the conflict. He concludes, however (p. 48), that the War was "worth more than it cost" if it was necessary for emancipation and for saving the Union.

[19] Livermore, *Numbers and Losses in the Civil War,* pp. 5–8.

[20] C. Vann Woodward, "The Irony of Southern History," *Journal of Southern History,* XIX (February, 1953), 4 f. Dr. Woodward quotes Professor Toynbee's remark that Americans in the North, like Englishmen, had no feeling by the 1890's that history had ever "happened" to them. True as this statement is, it again brings out the lapse of regional memory in the North. History, though forgotten, had indeed "happened" there in the loss of several hundred thousand men in four years—a type of tragedy which the English had never experienced.

Northern family which recalled the Civil War with much feeling. And this was my own household, which lost no lives but did witness the destruction of its home town by Confederate troops—some time before Sherman marched through Georgia. It was probably after such experiences, direct or vicarious, that families passed on memories and resentments unto the third and fourth generations. Descendants living in ruined areas, moreover, were constantly reminded of "the War" by poverty or other adverse consequences long after an older generation's sacrifice in lives had ceased to have personal meaning.

If we could recall the actual suffering of 1861–65, we might not so readily view the Civil War in terms of epic grandeur. In fact, however, there is now a disinclination to admit that anything so vital could have been unfortunate in the long run. This disinclination may be based in some cases on thoughtful analyses. But more often, one suspects, a pessimistic view is almost instinctively avoided because it would disturb national optimism and therefore must not be incorporated into our philosophy of history. Such an attitude may be detected today in the South as well as in the North, and it presumably inspires current "celebrations" of the Centennial.

We shall never know the final truths here, since no one can discover what would have followed if things had happened otherwise in 1861. Yet those who believe that the War was an ultimate triumph, alike with those who view it as ultimate tragedy, must base their conclusions on some calculus of might-have-beens. The former must assume that alternatives to war would have been worse in the final reckoning; the latter, that they would have been better.[21]

[21] An earlier discussion of this point is given in the author's "The Nationalistic Tradition of the Civil War," *South Atlantic Quarterly,* XXXII (July, 1933), 294–305; reprinted in part in *The Causes of the Civil War,* ed. Kenneth M. Stampp (Englewood Clifls, N.J., 1959), pp. 294–305.

This much seems reasonably certain: we should guard against the assumption that all major outcomes in the American past must have been for the best. Time may heal all things but does not necessarily justify them. With this thought in mind and recalling the medical story, one may still cherish doubts about what was called in some circles the War between the States. This, of course, was just what it was not. It was not a conflict among abstract "states" but rather a struggle between real men—with all the consequences which this entailed.

PERSONAL AND PUBLIC
HYGIENE

V

Sylvester Graham and
the Popular Health Movement,
1830-1870 *

It is impossible to foresee just what sort of immortality awaits one, either in this world or the next. Few would expect to have their names go down in history merely as labels for food and drink, yet this has been by no means a unique experience. The pathetic memory of a little English maid, the first of her race to be born in America, has been preserved chiefly in a trade name for wines and extracts. The time may come when Madame Melba will be remembered only because of her association with a concoction of peaches and cream. Sad as this may be, it seems less so than the fate of the leader of an interesting and important reform movement, who is recalled today—if recalled at all—only in connection with such prosaic foods as bread and crackers. Even "Peach Melbas" would seem to offer a more elegant avenue to posterity. Yet in a sense this was of the reformer's own choosing, and thereby hangs a tale.

Sylvester Graham began his career as a temperance lecturer in Pennsylvania in 1830.[1] Like the many idealists of the day

* Reprinted from the *Mississippi Valley Historical Review*, XVIII, No. 2, September, 1931—by permission.
[1] An early note on Graham's career will be found in the *Boston Medical and Surgical Journal*, XLV (1851), 316, and some biographical material is contained in his own *Æsculapian Tablets of the Nineteenth Century*

he was inspired, by a species of religious enthusiasm, to save mankind. While others were concerned with such matters as drink, women's rights, and the peace movement—wine, women, and war—Graham's distinction lay in the fact that he soon discovered, or at least believed that he had discovered, one more cause than had occurred to any of his colleagues. To put it plainly, he decided that the way to a man's salvation was through his stomach. The advance of an idealistic temperance reformer, to this apparently materialistic view was really quite a logical one. Why, he inquired of his associates, should temperance be limited to drink? After all, even the most thirsty could not live by liquor alone. Were not men made gross, even diseased, by intemperance in food as well? If drunkenness had slain its thousands, gluttony had certainly accounted for as many more.[2]

Physicians would probably agree that there was something in this idea. No one would dare estimate the exact degree to which earlier generations overate, but gormandizing was certainly one of their favorite indoor sports. Over-indulgence in meat and starches was particularly common, and has persisted in certain conservative sections, or among old-fashioned people, to this day. It may be that this "heavy" diet had been well adapted to the needs of pioneers, but its persistent popularity among their sedentary descendants was, to say the least, rather unfortunate. That it was generally popular is best attested by the amount of meat which was consumed. Historians who are wont to list the quantity of wine imbibed by

---

(Providence, 1834). The best biography is that by Mrs. George Genzmer, which will appear in a forthcoming volume of the *Dictionary of American Biography.*

[2] One of Graham's associates estimated that although alcoholism killed 50,000 Americans annually, "folly in dress" accounted for 80,000 while "downright gluttony" destroyed a round 100,000. Boston *Moral Reformer,* I (1835), 198.

sundry fathers of this country, might in addition remind us of their capacity for roasts and barbecues. An old cook book solemnly warned young husbands not to expect more than *three* sorts of meat, in case they brought the boys home to dinner unannounced. How many could be anticipated in case of a premeditated orgy was left to the imagination. The menus of ceremonial banquets, however, show that it was not unusual to serve as many as thirty or more kinds of meat and fish at one occasion. And leisurely ante-bellum gentlemen sometimes sat at the festive board for as much as seven hours at a stretch. Small wonder that gout and other ills were rather expected as the marks of good living.[3]

When this situation was fully realized by Graham it fired his spirit, even as the evils of slavery—real or imaginary—seared the souls of the abolitionists. Once aroused, he naturally discovered that the problem was an even more serious one than he had at first supposed. The American people were apparently headed straight for physical degeneracy.[4] Men not only suffered from bad habits connected with food and drink, but from many other violations of nature's "physiological laws." Here again it must be recalled that this generation rarely bathed, rarely opened a window, rarely (in the case of town dwellers) took any regular exercise, and in general lived in many respects much as poorer Europeans are pictured living today.

Consider the simple matter of bathing. For one thing, conditions of living did not encourage it. As Harriet Beecher

[3] For a detailed picture of such a feast, with its after effects, see Richard H. Shryock (ed.), *Letters of Richard D. Arnold, M.D., 1808–1876*, in Trinity College Historical Society, *Papers*, XVIII–XIX (Durham, 1929), 25, 26.

[4] It is to be remembered that there was also serious medical opinion to this effect; as that quoted in the Atlanta *Hygienic and Literary Magazine*, I (1860), 21.

Stowe pointed out, few could be expected to bathe *via* the old oaken bucket that hung in the well.[5] This was particularly true during the winter, when the water had to be heated before an open fire. The invention of stoves added to the comfort of the winter bath, but in cutting off the ample circulation afforded by the open fire places brought a problem of ventilation. However trying the ordeal, there was a real fear that winter bathing occasioned colds and other ills, whereas dirt was viewed as a sign of honest toil, plain living, and good health—the noble insignia of the common man. Even those who responded to Graham's appeals continued to have their doubts on this score. Thus one finds "a young man of great promise" remarking anxiously: "I have been in the habit during the past winter of taking a warm bath every three weeks. Is this too often to follow the year round?" [6]

Such an inquiry reveals a state of mind that was by no means peculiar. Daniel Drake, in his classic observations on the Mississippi Valley, solemnly declared that the people of this region seldom or never bathed.[7] Nor is there any reason to believe that effete easterners were much more civilized in this respect. In a word, Graham did not have to look far for bad habits without end. He therefore began to advocate not only a vegetarianism that included wholewheat products but also the virtues of bathing, fresh air, sunlight, dress reform, sex-hygiene, and exercise. By this time, the temperance ideal had obviously developed in his mind into something far more comprehensive; namely, the ideal of sensible living and good health in all its phases—of a sound body and a sound mind.

[5] Not only Mrs. Stowe, but Horace Greeley and other celebrities of the day became interested in hygienic reform. See Mrs. Stowe's interesting "Sermon on Your Health," *Atlantic Monthly*, XVIII (1865), 85 ff.

[6] Boston *Moral Reformer*, I (1835), 184.

[7] *Principle Diseases of the Interior Valley of North America* (Cincinnati, 1850), 679.

Personal hygiene was an old, old story,[8] but carrying it to the people with the fervor of a crusader was something relatively new. A request for the delivery of an address at the Franklin Institute in Philadelphia, in 1830, so encouraged Graham that he launched a series of lectures in New York and New England. Audiences numbering as many as two thousand persons attended and were apparently impressed.

Converts soon began sending in their testimonials. "Esteemed friend," wrote a Philadelphia Quaker, "I have been afflicted with frequent . . . severe head-ache. I attended thy course of lectures at the Franklin Institute last Spring and pretty strictly adopted the system of diet which thou didst recommend. . . . Since then I have been entirely free from head-ache and all other pains." [9] This sounds like the ordinary quack testimonial. Not so that of a subject who reported that he had been ruined by tea and coffee. "I decided," he declared "that I was in a decline. . . . At this time Mr. Graham commenced a course of lectures in New York. *I heard and trembled.* The torrent of truth poured upon me and made me a thorough convert. *But the coffee*—my greatest earthly comfort. My first effort to demolish the idol was on a Sabbath morning. *That* Sabbath will never be forgotten. A numbness and stupor came over me, and during the service I actually feared my rash resolve would cost me my life." After a bitter struggle and illness he finally redeemed himself from the curse of caffein.[10] Here, evidently, was a variety of religious experience overlooked by William James.

Graham eventually published nearly one hundred pages of these testimonials, a somewhat quackish procedure, but one he

[8] The first serious work on general hygiene published in this country was probably the edition of an English work (B. Grosvenor, *Health, An Essay on Its Nature,* etc.) which appeared at Boston in 1761.

[9] *Æsculapian Tablets,* 13.

[10] *Nature's Own Book* (New York, 1835), 52–54.

doubtless adopted with the best of intentions. As he himself pointed out, he had nothing to sell—his remedies "demanded no price." Meanwhile he gave primary attention to his lectures, which he wrote out at length, and eventually incorporated in his *Science of Human Health* [11]—a painstaking but verbose work, with a title which suggests one selected by a more famous health reformer of a later generation. Graham's work, however, was really scientific in the sense that it included the current physiology as well as hygiene; it having always been his contention that the latter must rest on a rational basis of "physiological principles." For this reason he became an ardent advocate of the popular teaching of physiology, and his followers were perhaps the first group to urge its introduction in the public schools.[12]

Groups of local disciples gathered in the wake of the lectures in New York and New England, where at that time any new form of social idealism was reasonably sure of sympathetic response. Women displayed a marked interest and special appeals were made to them. "Ladies' Physiological Reform Societies" began to meet for the discussion of "Grahamism" and to work for the general good of this new cause.[13] Mary Gove and Paulina Wright began to lecture to "female audiences"—a daring thing in itself—on hygiene and dress reform. In so doing they were even so brazen as to touch upon

[11] *Lectures on the Science of Human Health* (Boston, 1839).

[12] See the Boston *Health Journal and Advocate of Physiological Reform*, April 1, 1840. The later health cultists were also pioneers in demanding better light and air, as well as gymnastics in the schools. One group established a "Physiological School" at St. Anthony, Minnesota, in 1865, to serve as a model in such matters; New York *Herald of Health*, V (New Series, 1865), 153.

[13] Thus "The Ladies' Physiological Society of Millbury" subscribed to twelve copies of the Boston *Health Journal* in 1840, and distributed it throughout the town. "The ladies of this Society," explained the editor of that paper, "work at their meetings after the manner of charitable and anti-slavery societies. The sum earned is devoted to spreading information on health, and to the purchase of a Library."

anatomy and physiology, despite the consternation of the fair Victorians, who enlivened the lectures by a frantic search for salts and frequent faintings.[14] This crusade for women's health was related both in cause and effect to the demand for women's rights in general, and the health and feminist movements become indistinguishable at this point.[15]

Nor was there any neglect of the masculine world. "Graham boarding houses" were established in the larger cities, where the faithful of both sexes could observe the ritual already growing up within the cult; including the eating of "Graham bread" and the taking of a bath "in very warm water at least three times a week." At Brook Farm, a special table must needs be reserved for the Grahamites, to insure their proper diet; while in Boston a special bookstore was established to supply them with food for thought. In due time weekly papers were founded, bearing such appropriate titles as the *Graham Journal*, and the *Health Journal and Advocate*; and the "American Physiological Society" was established for the purpose of issuing appropriate tracts.[16]

These publications, which were instrumental in spreading

[14] Boston *Health Journal and Advocate*, April 1, 1840. Doris Stevens, of Washington, D.C., is authority for the note on Paulina Wright.

[15] It is presumably no accident that some of the earlier open appeals for birth control, in this country, appeared in the popular health journals; e.g., in the New York *Herald of Health*, VI (New Series, 1865), 97. It may be noted, in passing, that birth control seems to have been increasingly practiced in the United States from as early as 1840 on, opinion to the contrary notwithstanding. See William A. Alcott, *Physiology of Marriage* (Boston, 1856), 180; and Richard H. Shryock, "Public Relations of the Medical Profession," in *Annals of Medical History*, II (New Series, 1930), 327; and cf. C. V. Drysdale, "The Birth Control Movement After a Century's Agitation," *Current History*, XXX (1929), 382–83. On the origin of this movement in the United States, see Norman E. Himes, "Robert Dale Owen, the Pioneer of American Neo-Malthusianiam," *American Journal of Sociology*, XXXV (1930), 529 ff.

[16] Regular physicians also were sponsoring health periodicals during the period, as in the case of the Philadelphia *Journal of Health*, edited by Dr. D. F. Condie.

propaganda beyond the limits of the East,[17] were edited by leading disciples of whom the most active, Dr. William Alcott, displayed enthusiasms similar to those which characterized his cousin, Amos Bronson Alcott. Indeed Alcott and others were inclined to become more ecstatic about the cause than was Graham himself. The editor of the Boston *Health Journal* was of the opinion that

> among the numerous subjects of reform which are now engaging the attention of the community, those who are interested in physiological reform should not permit it to fall behind the others . . . for it is second to no other in importance—we believe it lies at the foundation of all others, and that wherever this is effected, there will the efforts of other reformers be most effectual. It is peculiarly suited to raise man from a state of sensual degradation and raise him to the rank, which as a rational and immortal being, nature intended he should occupy. . . . Will not those who feel for the present and everlasting welfare of their race, come to our aid? [18]

This, quite obviously, is not the language of a scientist lecturing on hygiene, but rather that of an idealist preaching salvation, albeit a moral and physical salvation instead of a theological one. The spirit of the Grahamites, like that of many reformers of their day, was that of a sublimated puritanism.[19]

[17] "The good cause is spreading here," wrote an Ohio correspondent, "people are inquiring and talking frequently, of . . . physiological reform. . . . I cannot keep my books at home." Boston *Health Journal and Advocate,* June 17, 1840.

[18] *Ibid.,* April 1, 1840.

[19] This is to be seen in the personal history of leaders, in the language used, in the enthusiasms displayed, and at times in the actual employment of theological arguments and conceptions. Thus Grosvenor, writing in the eighteenth century, declared health was essential to the next world as to this (*Health, an Essay,* etc., preface); while Asenath Nicholson argued that there was a physical as well as a moral "fall" in Eden, to be atoned for only by vegetarianism! (*Nature's Own Book,* 6.)

This spiritual kinship with contemporary idealists doubtless accounts for the gradual merging of Grahamism, after the leader's retirement in the 'forties, with similar movements which arose during this decade.[20] There was, in the first place, naturally some exchange of appreciation between perfectionists of all creeds,—the contact with the feminist movement has already been noted.

> We learn from the papers, [observed Alcott in 1835,] that the American Seventh Commandment Society, the New York Female Benevolent Society, the New York Ladies' Moral Reform Society, and the Anti-Tobacco Society, held their annual meetings at New York about the middle of May, and that some of these meetings were interesting.[21]

Despite such dubious praise it is evident that Alcott warmed to the members of these organizations as fellow seekers after light. On another occasion he noted the founding of flourishing anti-corset societies,—whose members "signed the pledge" not to wear them—and adds enthusiastically that "family associations" of this sort were numerous and increasing in number. More significant was the belief that "the disciples of Fourier and Graham" should work together.[22] Every good cause was sure of his moral support, even though there was not time for actual coöperation.

There was nothing tangible, however, in such diffuse appreciation of good works in general, and the Grahamites were soon to establish more immediate and vital contacts. In the course of lecturing on hygiene, Graham had naturally

[20] Not, however, until it had attracted such public attention as to elicit the compliment of a printed burlesque, wherein was described the debates of "the great American Society to Prevent Children Kicking off the Bed Clothes." This, it seemed, was organized to ponder the question "Suppose all the children would kick them off and take one universal cold, where would the nation be?" [Richard E. Selden], *The Newest Keepsake for Eighteen Hundred Thirty-Nine*, etc. (Boston, 1839), 17, 30.
[21] Boston *Moral Reformer*, I (1835), 225.
[22] Boston *Health Journal and Independent Magazine*, I (1843), 29.

asserted that right living was a more certain means to health than was a resort to doctors and drugs. It was but a step from this to the view that, if the laity would but practice hygiene, there would be no need for physicians to practice medicine. Graham himself never went quite that far but others were bound to carry his thought to a logical conclusion; hence Grahamism began to be viewed as a popular substitute for regular medicine. Anti-medical philosophy was characteristic of the day. Indeed, the popular protest against drugs and bleeding had been gaining headway for nearly a century before the Grahamites appeared upon the scene; and though at first haphazard, this protest finally began to take form about a number of medical heresies like homeopathy and "Thomsonianism." Just as these developed in response to the demand for a milder medication, so it may be said that Grahamism arose as a result of opposition to any medication whatever. In a word, the movement met the needs of its generation in both a positive and negative manner, positively, in its promotion of hygiene, negatively, in its avoidance of drugs.

The negative influence it shared, as was just noted, with several medical sects. Differing as these did in many respects, they agreed that the people must avoid the regular profession and all its wicked works. Their attack on the physicians was more successful than is generally realized today. All along the medical front, during the 'forties, the volunteer reformers pressed against the "regulars," and the latter in many places gave way. All American laws against irregular practice were gradually repealed or nullified, until anyone could be a "doctor" and practice as he pleased.[23]

Not the least energetic of the new sectarians were the hydropaths. The "water cure" (employed inside and out) was originally made in Germany, but reached America about

[23] Shryock, *op. cit.*, in *Annals of Medical History*, II, 322, 323.

1840. Though often cultivated by amateurs of the get-rich-quick variety, it assumed a quasi-respectability with the establishment of hydropathic institutes or "cures." Here various innovations were provided, such as the "Turkish Baths" introduced during the 'sixties, and a tendency was displayed to try anything once.[24] The chief genius of these early establishments seems to have been Dr. T. H. Trall, who expanded his "cure" in New York City into a general "hygienic institute," where he provided invalids with all manner of special treatment. Drugs were taboo, of course, as well as all other "regular" therapeutics, but to bathing he added diet, exercise, and electricity. He was, therefore, in entire sympathy with Dr. Dio Lewis, who began giving physical culture lessons in Boston during the early 'sixties, and one of whose pupils established a normal school of physical culture in New York City in 1865.[25]

During the 'seventies and the ensuing decades many other "cures" were established practicing what became known as the "hygienic system." Most of these were located in towns of the East and Middle West and a considerable number owed their origin to men trained by Trall.[26] Unusually successful ones appeared in Bloomington and Battle Creek, which places also became centers of publication as well, and from whence there issued in increasing numbers books, pamphlets, periodicals, and eventually "breakfast foods." In 1862 a "World's Hygiene Association" was founded in Chicago, and during the ensuing decade held sessions there and in New York City.

What Trall and his followers really did was to superimpose

[24] The first bath of this kind in America was said to have been opened in Brooklyn, in 1863. The introduction of these modern "Turkish Baths" in English-speaking countries is described in the New York *Herald of Health*, XLII (1892), 244, 245.

[25] *Ibid.*, V (New Series, 1865), 221.

[26] The local appeal and methods of such practitioners are described in their periodicals. See the *Herald of Health*, V (New Series, 1865), 166, for an example.

Grahamism upon hydropathy, and later, in the most catholic spirit imaginable, to add every other hygienic procedure available. Trall acknowledged his indebtedness to Graham and Preisnitz (Silesian founder of the "water cure"), but claimed to improve upon both. This latter-day health saint, unlike Preisnitz, became much more than an empiric; he elaborated a theory of disease (after the manner of the eighteenth-century physicians) and persuaded the New York legislature to incorporate a "medical school" connected with his institute. His progress from an empirical to a quasi-professional status is suggested by the changes made in the name of his paper. This publication which was probably the most successful of all the early health journals appeared regularly for some forty years, first as *The Water Cure Journal*, later as *The Herald of Health*, and finally as *The New York Journal of Hygiene*. Thus, by a process not unknown to medical historians, the sect became successful by approaching the standards of regular medicine. What should be emphasized, however, is that the latter also maintained itself by incorporating the best thoughts of the sect. The real debt of modern hygiene to these health reformers is seldom appreciated; the very principles for which Graham, Trall, and others fought—the danger of drugs, the importance of hygiene, and the ounce-of-prevention philosophy in general—were in due time largely accepted by the regular profession. It would seem that regular and sectarian ideas eventually merged in fact if not in form; medical developments thus following the order of thesis, antithesis, and synthesis.

The chief exceptions to this are to be noted in connection with the faddist fringe of the reformers' theories, as displayed in their views on vegetarianism or in their conviction that candy led directly to the grave. They trembled "to find the young so fond of . . . condiments and confectionaries." "There is no assurance," they felt, that those so enamored

"will not descend—and descend—till they arrive at the lowest
point of the scale of intemperance, gluttony and debauchery.
Even in female seminaries there is abundant cause for gloomy
anticipations." [27] One gathers that they rather relished these
"gloomy anticipations."

The most dubious phase of the reformers' work seems to
have been that relating to sex hygiene. Some of the health
faddists were probably active in the early "societies for
discouraging licentiousness," such as those organized in New
York, Boston, Hartford, Utica, "and many more places"
during the 'thirties. In these cities, long before the advent of
Anthony Comstock, little groups demanded "the indiscrimi-
nate punishment" of all "sellers of obscene prints" and the
like.[28] There was something very sane in Alcott's opinion that
such action would be "premature and of doubtful utility," but
he himself engaged in a campaign which was equally ques-
tionable. For it was he and certain associates who first told the
Americans at great length "what a young man should know."
Graham, Alcott, and Trall all wrote voluminously along this
line, and their work was apparently widely read in both the
United States and Germany.[29] This literature was originally
well intentioned and some of it may have been worth while.
Certainly no one would accuse them of such a deliberate

[27] Boston *Moral Reformer*, I (1835), 50–52.
[28] *Ibid.*, I, 33, 34.
[29] The interest of the later leaders in sex hygiene may have involved
both disinterested and mercenary motives; in any case it is worthy of
further study. Some of their many titles will suggest the character of the
literary tradition they established; e.g., Graham, *Chastity, in a Course of
Lectures to Young Men;* Alcott, *Young Man's Guide, Young Women's
Guide, Physiology of Marriage;* Trall, *Marriage and Parenthood, Mysteries
of Man,* etc. His *Home Treatment of Sexual Abuses* retailed at fifty cents,
in order that "it should be read by every young man in the land"; while
H. C. Wright's *Unwelcomed Child or the Crime of an Undesigned and
Undesired Maternity* could be had for seventy-five cents from the same
publishers. This last item suggests that there may have been a considerable
circulation of birth control literature earlier than is usually supposed to
have been the case; cf. Drysdale, *op. cit.,* in *Current History,* XXX, 383.

exploitation of sex as has characterized certain later popular health prophets. Yet in their semi-religious enthusiasm they exaggerated what was sweetly termed "American amativeness." Perhaps they thought to frighten youth into virtue by exaggerating the consequences of vice—a procedure already well tried in connection with the campaign against alcohol and tobacco. Or perhaps they simply exhibited that self-conscious fear of sex supposed to have characterized Victorians, and as a result of this really believed that all our youth were headed for the insane asylums,—just as they believed that all our drinkers were headed for the gutter.[30] In any case their rather unscientific propaganda must have been responsible for some harm, even so late as the beginning of the present century.

In the long run, however, the popular health movement accomplished good rather than ill. It has already been observed that physicians eventually accepted their general principles, though not simply because of the efforts of the reformers. Perhaps more important than this was the fact that the public came, to some extent, to apply these principles. A century after Graham first made his appeal, his preachments have begun to be practiced, and today at least part of the population apparently eat less and select their food with greater care than did their fathers. People nowadays are seekers after roughage and the whole grain in cereals. They worship fresh air and sun-tan, and the bath room has become the very symbol of American civilization. Verily, Americans have been "physiologically reformed."

[30] Typical expressions of this attitude may be found throughout the pages of the Boston *Health Journal and Advocate,* and the Boston *Moral Reformer.* (See the latter, I, 64.) It is only fair to note, however, that the reformers' exaggeration of the evils of sexual perversion reflected a similar though milder exaggeration in the medical literature of the day, which seems to have emanated from such continental authorities as Tissot, Bauer, etc. See Thomas Beddoes, *Hygeia,* I, 34 ff. (Bristol, 1802); and M. P. Tissot, *Oeuvres* (Paris, 1809), III, 248 ff., 291 ff.

All of this, it may be added, was not accomplished simply by the Grahamites, the water cures, the hygienic institutes, and the health journals. Such impersonal factors as mechanical improvements, scientific progress, and rising standards of living have made their contributions. Credit is also due to individuals and organizations among physicians, educators, and social workers in general. The fact remains that, at least in the earlier period, the popular health reformers were the most energetic and the most vocal of the groups mentioned—seemingly the only one which approached that degree of organization and enthusiasm necessary to the popularization of any cause. It would seem probable that they exerted a corresponding degree of influence in making possible the success of the whole movement. And it may also be assumed in conclusion that such success has meant much to our people in terms of esthetic values, decreasing illness, and even a lowered mortality rate; for a general improvement in personal hygiene is obviously an important factor in the improvement of the public health as a whole.

Graham and his followers, then, strove with some success to benefit their fellows, to aid not one kind of man but rather all mankind. The question at length arises whether they are not deserving of at least that measure of recognition which has been accorded their brothers in reform who sought to aid a particular class, or sex, or section? Yet the names of the latter appear on many a pedestal, while Graham's is still relegated to the grocery store.

VI

The Early American
Public Health Movement *

There has been some tendency, in recent years, to refer to the early public health movement as having been largely "a matter of pipes" or a campaign against smells. The subject seems literally as well as figuratively a trifle malodorous; and there is an inclination to pass over it hurriedly in order to consider the superiority of the public hygiene of our own day. All this would have seemed startling to those early public health leaders who, nearly a century ago, felt that they had already undertaken the great health reform of modern times. There was, for example, Wilson Jewell of the Philadelphia Board of Health who, before anyone had heard of Pasteur and Koch, believed that the new health epoch had arrived. As early as 1851, he planned a national public health association, and in 1857 he led in the actual establishment of such an organization. "Happily for the cause of humanity and the science of public health," he then declared, this body "has inaugurated a new era in the domain of science." [1]

Now one may well raise the question: By what process does a program once viewed as "a new era in the domain of science" descend in our memories to a mere "matter of pipes" or a campaign against smells? By a simple process of forget-

* Reprinted from *American Journal of Public Health*, Vol. 27, No. 10, October, 1937—by permission.

[1] Wilson Jewell, to John H. Griscom, Phila., Sept. 24, 1859; in *Proc., Third Nat. Quar. & Sanitary Convention* (New York, 1859), p. 5.

ting, perhaps—a natural result of the continuous pressure of present interests and present obligations. Yet this is neither good history nor, presumably, is it good for our souls. It is neither fair to the pioneer sanitarians nor to ourselves; for there is always the danger that indifference to the past will promote complacency in the present. It is therefore the purpose here to recall briefly the chief characteristics of the early American public health movement. "Lest we forget . . ."

The story relates chiefly to the three or four decades preceding 1870, although it has a background reaching far into the preceding centuries. The early industrial revolution along the American seaboard, as in Western Europe, made the problems of public health more striking and more obvious than they had ever been before. The city concentrated disease and misery, as the poorest rural areas could never do. Wherever one turned in the growing manufacturing and mercantile towns, there was the same picture. The American of 1840 read with horror of Scottish tenements, where whole families crowded into single rooms, were provided with no running water, and paid their rent by selling their own dung heaps accumulated in the courts below.[2] Yet at home, in New York City, more than half the population lived in similarly overcrowded tenements, and some 25,000 people occupied the damp and dismal cellars of these same buildings. In Cherry Street, to be specific, a five story tenement occupying only two ordinary building lots, housed 120 families, which included more than 500 individuals.[3] I say merely "individuals" for under such circumstances one can hardly speak of them as

[2] *Report on an Inquiry into the Sanitary Condition of the Labouring Population of Great Britain*, London, 1842, pp. 183 ff.

[3] *Proc.* cited above, pp. 523 ff. See also J. H. Griscom, *The Sanitary Condition of the Laboring Population of New York*, New York, 1845. For literature relating to other cities see R. H. Shryock, "Origins of the American Public Health Movement," *Ann. Med. Hist.*, n.s., I, New York, 1929, 658 ff.

"human beings." Similar conditions obtained in the slums of other American cities, and if it were desirable these could be described *ad nauseam.*

As might be expected, such circumstances made disease problems more acute as well as more obvious. The tragic history of the major endemic diseases, typhus, typhoid, and tuberculosis, is familiar enough. So far as can be judged from the imperfect bills of mortality, urban death rates rose ominously during the first half of the nineteenth century. New York City, which was most inundated by poor immigrants and which grew most rapidly, again affords a striking example. In 1810, the crude death rate had been reported as about 21 per 1,000; by 1857 it had risen to around 37—an increase of almost 80 per cent within 50 years.[4] Rates were lower in Philadelphia, but higher in New Orleans. What an increasing mortality implied in morbidity rates, to say nothing of "subclinical illness," is obvious enough.

Such conditions and such consequences cried to high heaven for reform. In both Europe and America a few socially minded physicians had long demanded improvements, but for some time they were unheeded. The public was apathetic: and under the growing spell of a *laissez faire* philosophy, the upper classes were inclined to let the poor shift for themselves. The latter died by the thousands, of unnecessary endemic diseases; and as long as their sufferings were not too obvious or did not threaten to spread to the better parts of towns, who cared?

What was evidently needed, in order to arouse the public conscience, was an epidemic which would dramatize disease and which would also threaten to spread it uptown.[5] Tubercu-

[4] Bolduan, C. F., "Over a Century of Health Administration in New York City," New York City Dept. of Health, *Mon. Ser.*, No. 13, Mar., 1916, p. 3; *Proc., Third Nat. Quar. & Sanitary Convention*, pp. 241, 523.

[5] Ravenel, M. P., "Endemic Diseases Versus Acute Epidemics," *A.J.P.H.*, 10:761 ff., 1920.

losis, which was becoming the great plague of the age, was of little service here, since it killed slowly, and the fear it aroused was in no way proportionate to its fatality. Smallpox was more promising, and likewise yellow fever; but the disease which best filled all the specifications was cholera. It struck at both town and country in the most mysterious, sudden, and fatal manner. The upper classes were not entirely spared, nor could they always escape observing the sudden collapse of the less fortunate. After this disease had passed, there was usually a demand for action.

A single illustration will suffice to show why this was so. When cholera visited Bishop Polk's Louisiana plantation in 1849, there were 350 Negroes there—shall we say, "in residence." Within two weeks, 220 contracted the disease, and no less than 70 died on this one place.[6] The conditions obtaining during such a "visitation" can scarcely be imagined, but it is a safe assumption that the Bishop felt that something should be done about it.

What could be done was none too clear. The disease moved like a contagion, but it struck hardest in slum areas or among the cabins of the poor. Those who maintained the seventeenth-century emphasis upon contagion demanded quarantine against cholera, but this signally failed to check its spread. On the other hand, the connection between the disease and bad living conditions was too obvious to be overlooked. Hence the experience with cholera weakened the hold of the contagion-quarantine doctrine and encouraged the revival of the classical thesis concerning airs, waters, and sanitary control. Those who feared cholera, or other epidemic diseases, now combined with humanitarians to demand investigations and clean-ups on a scale never demanded before. In these circum-

[6] Fenner, E. D. (ed.), *South. Med. Rep.*, New Orleans, 1:221, 259, 371 ff., 1850.

stances is to be found the genesis of the modern public health movement.[7]

The first stage in this movement was one of extensive investigation. Individual physicians had already shown the way here; notably in the case of Villermés' studies of 1828, in which he had shown that disease was to a considerable extent a result of living conditions throughout France. Similar observations were made during the '40's by Arnot and Kay in London, by Griscom in New York City, and by Virchow in Silesia. Meanwhile, Chadwick carried out his famous national survey for the Poor Law Board in England.

Since there were no national or state medical offices in the United States, surveys here could be carried out only by towns or by private organizations. The National Institute in Washington called for a wide investigation, but could secure no help from governmental authorities. It then turned to the American Medical Association, when that body was formed in 1847, and persuaded it to report on the sanitary conditions of large American cities. In consequence of its findings, the American Medical Association recommended to state and local medical societies the two procedures which seemed indicated under the circumstances: (1) that the registration of vital statistics, hitherto restricted to large towns, be undertaken by all the states in order that a clear picture of disease trends could be obtained; and (2) that sanitary reform should be pushed at once in urban and even in rural areas.[8]

State medical societies thereupon began appealing to their respective legislatures for registration laws. The American Statistical Association, founded at Boston in 1839 in response to the development of that branch of mathematics, also

---

[7] Shryock, R. H., *The Development of Modern Medicine*, Philadelphia, 1936, pp. 212 ff.

[8] *Trans.*, A.M.A., I:305–310, 1848; IV, 517 ff., etc., 1851.

supported this drive. Unfortunately, the extreme individualism and often the plain ignorance of democratic assemblies blocked such efforts in most American states—just at a time when progress was being made abroad. In Georgia, for instance, the legislature "fairly hooted" when a registration bill was introduced in 1849, and the whole matter was viewed as just another "trick of the doctors." [9] Yet Massachusetts did provide for state registration in 1843, and thus set an example which could thereafter be used in other states. Incidentally, as is well known, it thus provided for the longest mortality record of state population now available in this country.

The second part of the program urged by the American Medical Association; namely, actual sanitary reform, also made some progress during the decades before the Civil War. The early fear of yellow fever and of malaria had prompted some action in seaboard towns, even before the cholera epidemic emphasized this need. When yellow fever had devastated Philadelphia in the epidemics of 1793 and ensuing years, for example, the physicians who ascribed it to local filth persuaded the city to establish a permanent board of health. They also persuaded the town to clean up its streets, and to build one of the first free public water systems in the country. It should be noted that while Dr. Benjamin Rush and the others who insisted on the local origins of disease were partially wrong, their mistaken theories nevertheless had value in promoting urban improvements. It is also interesting to observe that, perhaps as a result of these developments, Philadelphia maintained a relatively low death rate and became known as "First in the cause of sanitary reform." [10]

Other cities followed this lead, between 1800 and 1850, in

[9] Shryock, R. H. (ed.), *The Arnold Letters*, Durham, N.C., 1929, pp. 36–39 (*Papers of the Trinity Col. Hist. Soc.*; Duke Univ., XVIII–XIX).
[10] Proc., *Third Nat. Quar. & Sanitary Convention*, pp. 680, 693.

establishing boards of health.[11] These boards were, to be sure, largely of an advisory nature and had no permanent health officers save for quarantine officials; but they provided the beginnings of a permanent organization which was expanded later when the need was finally recognized. For the time being their most common functions were to advise during emergencies, and to inspect premises for nuisances. There was little state law on medical police save with relation to licensing and quarantines, but city ordinances were passed in the tradition of the English common law on nuisances.[12]

Occasionally these boards were able to secure substantial sanitary improvements, which in turn were apparently successful in decreasing morbidity and mortality rates. A notable example is afforded in the case of Savannah. Here the death rate from "autumnal fevers"—chiefly malaria—was reported, early in the century, at the amazing average of 70 per 1,000. Assuming the airs and waters etiology, which for obvious reasons proved quite effective in this case, the city eliminated all wet culture of rice in the vicinity in 1818. The autumnal mortality thereupon fell to an average of 26 for the next 6 years, and declined even more during the ensuing period.[13]

This, to be sure, was an exceptional case. Most American towns were still lagging in sanitary improvements during the '50's, and it is rather startling to recall that places as large as Providence and Milwaukee then had no public water systems.[14] Faced by such inertia, and absorbed in difficult technical and professional problems, the American Medical Association apparently lost its first enthusiasm for sanitary

---

[11] The dates are given in J. M. Toner, Boards of Health in the United States, *Reports and Papers*, A.P.H.A., I:499 ff., 1873.

[12] Shryock, R. H., *Development of Modern Medicine*, pp. 86 ff., 241 ff.

[13] Gamble, Thomas, Jr., *History of the Municipal Government of Savannah, 1790–1901*, pp. 143 ff. (Included in The Mayor's *Ann. Rep.*, Sav., 1900.)

[14] Cole, A. C., *The Irrepressible Conflict*, New York, 1933, p. 181.

reform.[15] There seemed, in consequence, to be a need for some other organization to take up the leadership in health reform on a national scale. If the majority of physicians could not be interested in public hygiene, moreover, perhaps conscientious laymen could combine with socially minded doctors to set up a national health organization.

The answer to this need was found in the interesting national sanitary conventions that met from 1857 to 1860, and which began to function as the first association in America definitely devoted to the study of public health. Wilson Jewell, who was mentioned above, saw in the meeting of an international quarantine conference in Paris a suggestion for an analogous interstate meeting in this country. State quarantine regulations varied as much as did those of different nations, and merchants as well as medical men regretted the confusion involved. Jewell called the first meeting at Philadelphia in 1857, and municipal officials and doctors from the chief Atlantic and Gulf ports responded.[16] Subsequent sessions were held in Baltimore, New York City, and Boston.

Although the conventions had ostensibly met to consider quarantine regulations, it was immediately apparent that the members were more concerned with "internal hygiene" (sanitation) than with the "external" form (quarantine). The advocates of the latter procedure were on the defensive from the start. Contagion was never entirely denied, notably in the case of smallpox, but the majority felt that the medieval doctrine had been greatly overdone—to the serious discomfort of both passenger and mercantile interests. Dr. Arnold, the

---

[15] On the early relation of the A.M.A. to public health reform, see *Proc., Third Nat. Quar. & Sanitary Convention*, p. 213; H. I. Bowditch's statement to the Intern. Med. Cong., Phila., 1876 (*Public Hygiene in America*, Boston, 1877, p. 37); Stephen Smith's "Remarks," *Papers and Reports*, A.P.H.A., XXII:21, 1897.

[16] *Minutes, Nat. Quar. & Sanitary Convention* (Philadelphia, 1857), pp. 3–11; *Proc., Third Nat. Quar. & Sanitary Convention* (New York, 1859), pp. 3–6.

mayor of Savannah and a delegate to the fourth convention, ridiculed the few contagionists, by recalling an occasion when his "excellent old aunt had been quarantined at New York because she had the gout." He concluded by thanking God that the conventions had "swept away one of the last relics of barbarism—the infernal restrictions of quarantine." [17]

The last stand of the contagionists was attempted during the discussions over yellow fever. Since physicians lacked as yet most laboratory technics, the empirical evidence on the causes and carriage of this disease was most confusing. Dramatic indeed were the yellow fever debates at the New York meeting, which subsequently filled more than 100 pages of the proceedings. Dr. Francis of New York, a gentleman of the old school, held to the early view that he had inherited from Dr. Hosack at the beginning of the century; namely, that "a contagious principle lurks in the fever now under discussion," [18] but the younger men overwhelmed him with evidence that it was never transmitted by contact—it was never a "man to man" affair. We can now see that both interpretations were right, and both wrong—a possibility that never seems to have occurred to either side in the controversy.

Having silenced the contagionists, the sanitarians next laid down their own program. This was somewhat broader than is now usually recalled, as it included not only model laws providing for state and local health boards, sanitary regulations, and modified quarantine laws, but also provided for experimental studies of sewage, ventilation, and disinfectants, and for the passage of pure food and drug laws. In a word, the delegates were concerned with research as well as with improved administration, and were as anxious to encourage the one as the other.

[17] *Proc., Fourth Nat. Quar. & Sanitary Convention* (Boston, 1860), p. 127.

[18] *Proc., Third Nat. Quar. & Sanitary Convention,* pp. 150 ff.

Last but not least, the members of the conventions were alive to the need of educating the public, although this is now often viewed as a "recent" function of health administration. To this end, they encouraged the formation of "sanitary associations" in large cities, similar to the "health of towns" societies in Great Britain. An apparently flourishing association of this sort, set up in New York City before 1860, was active in the drive which finally led to the reform of health administration in the metropolis.

In this connection, also, it should be recalled that the sanitarians were teaching the public a naturalistic as opposed to a theological or superstitious etiology. The concept of filth as a cause of disease was a bit vague, but it was actually more tangible than even the bacteria about which the public is now so generally informed. No wonder that sanitarians scoffed at superstitious fears, and that for prophylaxis they recommended clean-ups rather than fasts.

The efforts of the convention leaders to establish their association permanently seem rather pathetic, in view of the aftermath. Jewell wrote, in 1859, that he viewed the conventions as a permanent institution "destined to revolutionize the public mind and will." The Boston meeting of June 1, 1860, heard a discussion of plans for permanent organization, and appointed a committee to submit such plans at Cincinnati in 1861.[19] Enthusiasm was growing, and all looked forward to rapid progress in the immediate future. It was true that sectional tension along the Mason and Dixon line was increasing, but medical leaders ignored the political hubbub in Baltimore and points South. Arnold, of Savannah, presided at

[19] *Proc., Fourth Nat. Quar. & Sanitary Convention*, pp. 8, 13, 155. I am indebted to Dean Stanhope Bayne-Jones, of Yale University, for the proper emphasis upon the influences making for a naturalistic view of disease causation. In the paragraph above, however, I have projected his interpretation of the work of bacteriologists into the earlier efforts of the sanitarians as well.

the last sessions, and when he concluded with gracious praise of Boston hospitality, his New England hearers gave three cheers for Georgia! [20] That was about the last time that Arnold saw any Northerners, until he surrendered his city to Sherman's army one December day four years later. Such contrasts almost make one wish that the country had been governed by the doctors rather than by the politicians.

The outbreak of the Civil War in April, 1861, preceded the proposed Cincinnati meeting, and so the first national association came to an untimely end. Space does not permit a discussion of the diversion of public health endeavors into military channels; although this story is in itself an interesting one. Broadly construed, it includes such phases as the expansion of the Federal and the Confederate Medical Corps, the establishment by Dorothea Dix of the first trained nursing service in the United States base hospitals,[21] and, most important, the development of the U.S. Sanitary Commission.[22] That the war presented problems of public health on a peculiar scale will be obvious, when it is recalled that during the first year, five-sixths of the deaths in the Union armies were due to illness having no connection with the battlefields.[23]

The war also wrote other chapters in the history of disease and public hygiene which can be only mentioned here. There was the destruction of Southern economy and the consequent surging of ignorant rural Negroes into towns, where they gave up the crude health insurance provided by the slave system and in exchange received freedom and complete neglect. Thereafter, they indulged unhindered in life, liberty, and the

---

[20] *Ibid.*, p. 107.

[21] Marshall, Helen E., *Dorothea Lynde Dix* (Chapel Hill, N.C., 1937), pp. 201 ff.

[22] Stillé, C. J., *History of the U.S. Sanitary Commission* (Philadelphia, 1866), chaps. 1–3.

[23] *U.S. Sanitary Comm. Doc.*, No. 46 (New York, 1862), pp. 5 ff.

pursuit of the venereal diseases. Negro mortality rates rose rapidly above the white, after 1864; [24] and it is hardly exaggeration to say that only within the most recent years have some of the resultant problems been seriously attacked by the American government.

Incidentally, the war did some good—in spite of itself, one is tempted to say. Army medicine is state medicine by definition, and numbers of promising young men like John S. Billings and S. W. Abbott attained their early interest in public hygiene as a result of army experience. Older leaders also carried on in the same field; and after the war, picked up their sanitary reform program where they had dropped it in 1860. This was easier to do in the victorious North than it was in the devastated South. In 1869 Massachusetts finally provided for the State Board of Health which Shattuck had so well planned some twenty years before. And within three more years, a renewed call for a national body resulted in the formation of the present American Public Health Association. The somewhat jerky continuity of this story is illustrated by the fact that Dr. Elisha Harris of New York was one of the leaders in the early Sanitary Conventions, then served as an important member of the U.S. Sanitary Commission, and finally became the Secretary of the new American Public Health Association in 1872.

Another illustration will be found in the case of Dr. Arnold, the presiding officer of the Boston convention already mentioned. During the war he was in charge of a Confederate base hospital at Savannah; and then, in 1872, he accepted enthusiastically the invitation to join the revived public health association. As Arnold had also served as the first secretary of the American Medical Association, it is interesting to find him declaring—in these later years—that he had long considered

[24] See, *e.g.*, Duncan, W., *Tabulated Mortality Record of the City of Savannah* (Savannah, 1870), p. 36.

that organization a failure. He now pinned his hopes rather on the American Public Health Association.[25]

It is doubtful if many of those who organized this Association in 1872 could have had any realization of the great changes in public hygiene which lay just ahead of them. To their minds, they were picking up an old but promising movement for sanitary reform.[26] Now, however, as we look back upon them, the founders of the Association seem to have been inaugurating the new era that was ushered in by the bacteriological revolution.

That this revolution profoundly changed the nature of public hygiene is obvious to all. How effectively this was done is well recorded in the essays published by this Association in 1921.[27] Public hygiene entered a new and far more promising era in 1872. But for this reason, the present generation can afford to be generous in recalling the labors and achievements of those ante-bellum leaders who now appear to us as pioneers.

[25] Arnold to Dr. Elisha Harris, Savannah, April 26, 1873, in R. H. Shryock (ed.), "Selections from the Letters of R. D. Arnold," *Bull. Johns Hopkins Hosp.*, XLII:238, 1928.

[26] Note the nature of the papers and reports submitted to the Association between 1873 and 1876, as summarized in Stephen Smith's Historical Sketch of the A.P.H.A., *Reports and Papers*, A.P.H.A., V (Boston, 1880), XI ff.

[27] Ravenel, Mazÿck P. (ed.), *A Half Century of Public Health*, New York, 1921.

VII

The Historical Significance
of the Tuberculosis Movement *

On this occasion of the fiftieth anniversary of the first
American tuberculosis association—founded here in Philadelphia in 1892—the Committee on Archives and History
respectfully invites attention to the past. We suggest that the
members of the National Association turn aside for the
moment from immediate concerns and, as it were, ascend the
historical heights from which one can survey the path trav-
ersed by the tuberculosis movement during the last half
century. Only by thus looking back can we fully realize the
direction in which this national health organization has been
and is now moving. In order to achieve an historical perspective, the Committee has assembled the exhibits here on
display, and has also planned the papers to be delivered at the
present session. These arrangements are illustrative of the two
chief purposes of the Committee: first, the collection of all
types of records which otherwise may soon be lost; and,
second, the interpretation of such records in formal papers and
narratives. Such an historical presentation should not only be
of interest to those active in the National Tuberculosis
Association, but may also aid in demonstrating the significance
of the Association to the educated public as a whole.

* Reprinted from the *Transactions of the Thirty-eighth Annual Meeting
of the National Tuberculosis Association, 1942*—by permission.

Our interest in submitting a survey of the past half century is not only in the history of tuberculosis as a disease, nor in the technical medical problem it has presented. We are concerned rather with the fusion of these two phases of the story with a third; namely, with the development of a special public health society and its program. It therefore seems logical, before attempting the survey, to recall very briefly those circumstances which had to be realized *before* such an organization could be conceived or its program inaugurated. Some of these circumstances were social, others scientific in nature.

One would naturally assume, to begin with, that a prime condition of any movement against a given disease would be the actual existence of that disease in society. On second thought, however, this appears doubtful. Crusades were actually launched, in earlier days, against disorders which were largely the imaginary creations of the crusaders. In the sixteenth and seventeenth centuries, for example, a widespread drive against illness caused by black magic was undertaken in Europe and America. We now refer to this scornfully as the "witchcraft persecutions," but in the minds of contemporaries it partook of what we would today term a public health program. It died gradually as men lost faith in a theological prophylaxis.

Those devoted now to the extermination of tuberculosis need hardly fear that the ground will be taken out from under them by a denial of the reality of the disease. Unless society should revert to some superstitious philosophy, it will continue to view the existence of the white plague as all too real—either as an entity in itself or at least as a distinct "clinical picture." This suggests, however, one of the undoubted prerequisites we have in mind. The disease must be identified, and the more specific the identification the greater likelihood of an effective drive against it. It is no accident that most of the early, confused campaigns against a particular plague were directed towards skin diseases such as leprosy, syphilis, and smallpox—for the simple reason that skin conditions could be easily recognized by symptoms alone. Effective control of such *hidden* conditions as typhoid fever, on the other hand, had to await the development of modern pathology and bacteriology, before the infection could be fully identified and therefore specifically inhibited. Tuberculosis lay midway between these two types; it was vaguely known as a clinical picture through the ages, but even the pulmonary form was not clearly envisaged until modern pathologists correlated symptoms with lesions, and so were able to distinguish it from other pulmonary disorders. This research was not completed until the early nineteenth century, and it is obvious that no very effective public effort could have been directed against the disease until its specific identity had been so established.

Even the clear-cut recognition of a pathological entity, however, will not in itself insure public defense measures. For this is simply a scientific factor, and must be supplemented by social forces if widespread reactions are to come into play. Most potent of such forces is public fear. As is well known, a disease may be deadly enough and yet cause little alarm. Each disorder produces its own social psychology, in which mortality is at most only one of several variables. Best calculated to arouse fear are (1) suddenness and violence of attack, as in cholera, (2) mystery as to cause or transmission, as once in cholera and today in poliomyelitis, (3) obvious lingering symptoms or lesions, as in leprosy, smallpox, or poliomyelitis. Hence leprosy and cholera were ideally suited to arouse health drives. Conversely, a condition like nephritis, for all its mortality, produces almost no general fear at the present time.

Tuberculosis, unfortunately, was not calculated to produce hysteria. The onset was slow and there were at first no startling, visible lesions. Such symptoms as did appear—pallor or emaciation—were actually considered rather fascinating in early Victorian days, when a perverted sentimentality lingered lovingly over the young lady "going into a decline." It is too bad that humans did not wear their lungs inside out as do certain species of amphibians, for in such a case the concern aroused might have demanded some sort of protection. As it was, we owe to cholera and yellow fever, rather than to tuberculosis, the actual advent after 1800 of the first real public health efforts in this country.

Another social prerequisite to well organized disease drives was what might vaguely be termed a reform complex. Any society which, like that of medieval Europe, possessed little or no concept of progress, was not likely to organize programs for social betterment. One can speak of the medieval campaign against leprosy, but this was hardly an organized movement in the modern sense. Medieval men struck savagely at immediate dangers when these were apparent, but they were not motivated by any belief in continuous, long-run control. It was probably the impact and promise of modern science which produced the optimism of the eighteenth-century enlightenment, which in turn inspired the many reform movements which followed. By 1850 there was hardly any social evil in America which had not become the subject of a reform drive. Some of these now seem extreme or silly in retrospect. "We learn from the papers," observed Dr. William Alcott in 1835, "that the Seventh Commandment Society, the New York Female Benevolent Society, the New York Ladies' Moral Reform Society, and the Anti-Tobacco Society, held their annual meetings at New York about the middle of May, and that some of these meetings were interesting." But these were only the extreme fringe of great reform campaigns like the temperance, the anti-slavery, and the women's-rights upheavals, and not the least among the latter was the organization of the first American public health association in the 1850's.

It is interesting to observe, however, that this early public

health group that met in annual, so-called "National Sanitary
Conventions," gave practically no thought to tuberculosis. It
had a distinctly social motivation and, like the contemporary
"Health of Towns" societies in England, brought lay and
medical leaders together in a conscious effort to fuse social
and scientific facilities towards a common end. To this degree,
it was a prototype of the National Tuberculosis Association.
But it did not even recognize tuberculosis as having the status
of a health problem. The disease was now identified and there
was a slowly growing fear in terms of particular cases, yet it
was still entirely a private, individual alarm. I once read all the
correspondence of the last presiding officer of these conventions, Dr. Richard Arnold of Savannah, over a forty-year
period from 1835 to 1875. He was much concerned with
cholera and yellow fever as public dangers, but never referred
to "consumption" as such in all that time. Yet during the 40's
his own wife was slowly dying of this disease, and there were
many poignant references to the tragedy in the letters. In a
word, this public reformer harbored in his own home an
expression of the major health problem of the age—as we
would now term it—and never even recognized it. How can
one account for this apparent blindness?

The answer lies obviously in the lack of another scientific
prerequisite to a health drive against a specific disease. No
such effort can be attempted until it is felt that something can
be done about a disease danger, and here again science had to
supply the answer. Men could enter with enthusiasm on an
attack against yellow fever, because they at least thought they
could prevent it by quarantines or sanitary reform. But there
was no weapon at hand against tuberculosis. True, Dr.
Benjamin Rush had announced about 1800 his discovery that
it could be cured by the use of opium and an animal diet; but
the more critical outlook of the physicians of 1850 had long
made them skeptical of such earlier claims. "Consumption,"
then, belonged to that appalling legal category known as "an

act of God," and one does not undertake reform drives against the Deity.

The point of all this is clear enough. The advent of an antituberculosis movement had to wait, finally, upon the discovery of some means to prevention or cure. The first sign in this direction was the growing belief that a regimen of rest, diet, and fresh air held definite therapeutic possibilities, and the early sanatoriums appeared in consequence. More significant, but moving in the same direction, was the work of Koch and other bacteriologists, which itself would have been impossible without the earlier labors of the pathologists. The actual discovery of the tuberculosis bacillus, in terms of Henle's postulates, involved two outstanding achievements; first, a still more specific identification of the disease in relation now to etiological as well as to pathological phenomena; and, second, a prospect of more adequate prevention, if not of actual cure, in terms of the same etiological factor. The first made possible a clearer recognition of infection in non-pulmonary tissues, as well as in non-humans; the second motivated the whole campaign against means of transmission. Supplemented by the continued sanatorium program, these measures rather suddenly provided the weapons that could now be taken up in an organized tuberculosis drive. Again it was no accident that such a movement got under way in the years immediately following Koch's achievements.

Summing up, then, one can see how the historical stage was set so that the present National Association could play its striking rôle. No one factor was sufficient. All the elements mentioned—disease identification, the discovery of cause and consequent means of prevention, the slow growth of public fear and of a social reform psychology—contributed their part to a social-scientific ensemble out of which grew a great health association.

Last but not least, this body was fortunate in possessing far-seeing and able leaders who, in pioneer days, were able to make the most of the necessary social setting. Taking advantage of new scientific understanding and of other ideas seeping in from Europe, they built what was in many ways a new type of social institution. True, certain elements thereof had been earlier employed. The principle of a national health organization, and even of lay-medical cooperation, had been realized on a small scale in the "sanitary conventions" of the 'fifties. The scheme of a federal establishment, with interrelated local, state, and national societies, had been followed for some time by the American Medical Association. But the idea of focusing a national movement on a single, major disease was a novel one, and the specificity of this approach proved to have social as well as scientific advantages. Although the public had been slow to realize the threat of tuberculosis for all the reasons noted, it could be enlisted in a campaign against this one definite danger more readily than it could against so vague a concept as disease in general. The famous Christmas Seal sales brought an unprecedented response, and provided a financial foundation on which to build a program of remarkable proportions.

This success naturally led to emulation, and the Association became the prototype of other American societies with which we are all familiar, each of which has been devoted to the control of a particular disease. But none of these attained the significance of the National Tuberculosis Association. Nor did European organizations develop on the same scale. The story of the actual achievements of the Association, in relation to declining morbidity and mortality during the years since 1890, involves statistical and other types of interpretation which it is beyond the present purpose to consider. But even the most critical would agree that the activities of the Association greatly influenced the improvements in public health which so distinguished the recent era.

THE MEDICAL PROFESSION

VIII

The American Physician in 1846 and in 1946

A Study in Professional Contrasts *

Centenary celebrations afford a natural occasion for comparisons of the old and the new. The century which has elapsed since the Northern Medical Association of Philadelphia was founded in 1846 was one in which most aspects of civilization changed with unprecedented rapidity, and medicine was no exception to this rule. Hence the contrast between the status and activities of the American physician in 1846 and in 1946 involves much that may seem unusual to the modern observer.

The glance backward may also reveal some things which are of more than antiquarian interest, for certain problems persist even through a century of change. The most commonly aired grievance of American physicians during the 1840's, for example, was the difficulty of collecting fees. "It runs me almost crazy," wrote a successful practitioner about 1840, "to think that with hundreds upon hundreds due me professionally I find the greatest difficulty in raising a simple fifty dollars." [1] No doubt there has been improvement in this

* Reprinted from *The Journal of the American Medical Association*, May 31, 1947, Vol. 134, pp. 417–424. Copyright, 1947, by American Medical Association—by permission.

[1] Shryock, R. H.: *Letters of Richard D. Arnold, First Secretary of the American Medical Association*, Trinity College Historical Society Papers 18–19, Durham, N.C., Duke University Press, 1929, p. 21.

respect; but rumor has it that even now there is occasionally some difficulty of this sort, and the whole matter of professional income is involved in current discussions of health insurance. The earlier experience of members of the medical profession with this or with any other persistent problem invites comparisons which may throw light on contemporary situations.

Many who contemplate the past—and who does not do this occasionally?—go to one of two extremes. Some accept uncritically the modern faith in progress and assume that everything was pretty backward until they came along, while others reverse this attitude and succumb to a nostalgia for the good old days. In 1925 a Maine physician wrote this inquiry: "I wonder if the medical man is held in as high esteem, or is as important a factor in the community, as was his confrère a half century ago?" The reply was a negative one: the questioner was convinced that the doctor of 1875 had much the better position.[2]

For a real answer to his inquiry, of course, one must examine the evidence. A wealth of material immediately appears, pointing in the opposite direction. Whether one sticks to the 'seventies or goes back to the 'forties makes little difference, for a definite improvement in the status of members of the American medical profession did not set in until almost 1900. There were no public opinion polls then, by which to measure attitudes toward a profession; but the difficult position of physicians may be easily illustrated by random references. The newspapers of the 'forties and 'fifties, for example, sometimes ridiculed medical students and medical practice. Occasionally they went to extremes of condemnation. Thus the Philadelphia *Item* denounced (1858) the "poisoning and surgical butchery" which were common in

[2] Mann, F. W.: "The Public Status of Our Profession," *J. Maine M. A.,* 16: 137, 1925.

practice,[3] while in the next year a large daily paper declared that the whole medical guild was "a stupendous humbug." [4] Many lay critics had as low an opinion of professional behavior as they had of professional skill. "It has become fashionable," declared the editor of the *Cincinnati Medical Observer* during the 'fifties, "to speak of the Medical Profession as a body of jealous, quarrelsome men, whose chief delight is in the annoyance and ridicule of each other." [5] Alarmed by such attitudes, physicians had begun in the 'thirties to deliver addresses on "The Present Position of the Medical Profession." Two decades later they employed such frankly discouraged headings as: "To What Cause Are We to Attribute the Diminished Respectability of the Medical Profession in the Estimation of the American Public?" [6]

It is clear, after even such casual glances at the record, that all was not well with the profession a century ago. Granting that there still may be some cynicism about medicine, it is hard to imagine a daily paper referring to current surgical intervention as mere "butchery," or condemning professional practice as "a stupendous humbug." Compare with these epithets, for example, the respectful manner in which both contemporary newspapers and movies usually deal with physicians. About a decade ago there was a series of films which portrayed medical personnel in almost glamorous colors. These were embellished with such titles as "Men in White," "Women in White," "The White Parade" and so on. For a while anything "in white" was good for boxoffice returns. There were also such laudatory pictures as "Pasteur" and "The Magic Bullet," to say nothing of the late lamented "Dr.

---

[3] Philadelphia City *Item*, Nov. 6, 1858.

[4] M. & S. *Reporter*, 1: 356, 1859.

[5] Editorial, *Cincinnati M. Observer*, 2: 129, 1857.

[6] Editorial, M. & S. *Reporter*, 1: 141, 1859. There were many other such titles; Bauer, L.: "On the Declining Relations of the Medical Profession to the Public," *Cincinnati M. Obs.*, 2: 97, 1857.

Kildare." If Hollywood is to be trusted, the medical profession has today a far higher position in public esteem than it did in great-grandparents' days.

To what circumstances may one attribute the uncertain status of physicians a century ago? There is no one simple answer to this, any more than there is a single explanation of professional prestige at the present time. Various factors must be noted, if one is to understand the position in which physicians found themselves at the time this association was founded.

In an analysis of the status of any profession, one first thinks of the original process by which personnel is selected. One envisages today the years of college education and the standards of grade A medical schools, all of which tend to prevent the lazy or incompetent student from taking the Doctor of Medicine degree. But in 1846 almost any man with an elementary education could take a course of lectures for one or two winters, pass an examination and thereby automatically achieve the right to practice medicine by state law. Since the old training under an experienced physician (preceptor) had been gradually abandoned, doctors could be turned out in less than a year. As late as 1900 there were medical schools which admitted students who could not gain entrance to a good liberal arts college. To be sure, some college graduates went to the better medical schools; but a study made at Yale in 1850 indicated that most graduates preferred law and theology, and that those who did enter the field of medicine were usually not of high standing in their classes.[7]

It would be of interest to inquire, in passing, whether the first women to secure medical education were of superior caliber. One might expect this, in view of the opposition they had to overcome. Most physicians and laymen were shocked at

[7] Hooker, W.: "Report of the Committee on Medical Education," *Tr. A.M.A.,* 4: 409, 1851.

the very thought of a "doctress"; but after the Woman's Medical College was opened in Philadelphia in 1850 some newspapers encouraged the idea, and there was occasional support even in the medical journals.[8]

Whatever standards were maintained by the few "female" colleges, most schools admitted youths without higher education and with uncertain secondary school backgrounds. In 1854 a candidate requested admission to the Savannah Medical College on the impressive ground that he was proficient in the use of his own language. A professor in reply said that it would help if the student also knew something of the classics but added hastily that he could pick this up "with perfect ease" while attending the lectures. The student was invited to enter and reminded that he could not find a better college in that part of the country.[9]

This last remark was significant. The Savannah College was apparently a proprietary school, even though a superior one, and the practitioners who owned it needed the tuition fees. By 1850 the original university schools were pressed by the competition of proprietary institutions that sprang up all over the country. This proliferation has been ascribed to the increase of population and the consequent demand for more practitioners than the old schools could supply. But since the country already seemed oversupplied with physicians by the 'fifties other influences must have been at work. The late Dr. William H. Welch believed that the English medical schools (without university connections) set a bad example here. But the London schools were at least associated with hospitals, while American institutions sometimes lacked this advantage. The truth is that there was money in a successful medical college, since the owners maintained it simultaneously with

[8] Shattuck, G. C.: *The Medical Profession and Society,* Boston, D. Clapp & Son, 1866, p. 29.
[9] Shryock,[1] p. 68.

their private practice. The lower the standards, outside a few main centers, the higher were the registration figures and the profits. No wonder that schools multiplied, and that intense jealousies developed between the members of rival medical faculties.

Competition from mediocre schools hurt even the better institutions. When Pennsylvania tried to raise its entrance and course requirements during the 'forties, many youths were reported to be leaving for "easier quarters." The editor of the *Item*, already quoted, declared that even the Philadelphia students were coarse, crude and ignorant; a New York paper added the adjective "licentious" in describing the young medicos of that city.

Due allowance may be made for editorial exaggeration in such statements. But since they were supplemented by ample testimony from leading medical practitioners themselves, it is clear that the recruitment of the members of the profession was a rather casual process. This was of grave concern to professional leaders, and their efforts to form state medical societies were motivated in part by the effort to reform medical education. This was desired not only to provide better training per se but also to overcome the jealousies of rival schools. The same motives inspired the founding of the American Medical Association in 1847.[10] The national body encountered great difficulties, however, in seeking reform. Influential practitioners throughout the country were interested in proprietary schools and opposed standards which would have eliminated them. When Oliver Wendell Holmes, for example, condemned what he termed "inferior schools, wrongly located," he raised a storm throughout the South and West. Medical professors in those areas viewed this as a sectional attack on

[10] Fishbein, M.: "History of the American Medical Association," *J.A.M.A.*, 132:637 (Nov. 16) 1946.

themselves and ridiculed Holmes's "highfalutin' Boston notions."

Tied in with low standards in the schools was the general laxity of state licensing laws. Early in the nineteenth century certain states had enacted fairly good statutes, which provided for examination by state medical societies or boards. But it proved simpler to license automatically all who graduated from the schools; and as the latter deteriorated, licensing became almost a farce. Some reformers advocated federal licensure,[11] while others considered that the M.D. degree had become meaningless and urged that it be replaced for able men by some such designation as M.A.M.A. (Member, A.M.A.).[12] This would not control licensing, but would at least indicate the real physicians. Such protests achieved little until almost the end of the century, when the impact of scientific progress enabled the national Association to initiate a really effective reform movement.[13]

Another problem which faced medical societies a century ago was the relation of one practitioner to another. After the student had taken his degree, such as it was, he found himself in sharp competition on entering practice. By 1860 there was 1 practitioner for every 572 persons in the population as a whole. The ratio was apparently higher in rural than in urban areas—just the reverse of the present situation. The rural physician was then in great demand and suffered few such disadvantages as he does at present. In the North (relatively urban) there was 1 physician to 534 inhabitants; in the South, 1 to 526, and in frontier states, 1 to every 417. The general

[11] *New York J. Med.*, 5: 415, 1845.
[12] Sponsored by the New Jersey State Medical Society in 1858; M. & S. *Reporter*, 1: 283, 1859.
[13] The detailed story of medical education before 1860 is given in Norwood, W. F.: *Medical Education in the United States Before the Civil War*, Philadelphia, University of Pennsylvania Press, 1944.

average of 1 to 572 may be compared with that of 1938, which was 1 to 764.[14] The excess of physicians was such that many young graduates failed to secure a decent practice and abandoned the profession. The pressure of competition not only caused bitterness against sectarians but also created friction within the regular profession.

Prior to about 1800 there had been no rules to the game, and physicians even condemned one another in the newspapers. A famous illustration of professional friction in Philadelphia had been Benjamin Rush's newspaper debate with colleagues over the best methods of treating yellow fever. Laymen took sides, and in the course of this debate one critic referred kindly to Rush's method as "one of those great discoveries which are made from time to time for the depopulation of the earth." [15] Rush denounced his colleagues, resigned from the College of Physicians and viewed himself as a much-abused figure. This was typical of many professional quarrels.

These difficulties were not to be entirely explained by the competitive factor. This affected lawyers and business men as well, yet physicians were notorious for the peculiar rancor of their quarrels. Perhaps the vital nature of medical work made for unusual bitterness between rivals. Many a doctor, at a time when medicine was much more of an art than a science, honestly believed that competitors were killing their patients rather than curing them. Or, if the rival was not actually liquidating his clientele, he was doubtless doing them no good

---

[14] Eighth Census (Washington, D.C., 1850), pp. 670 and 677; cited by Stern, B. J.: "American Medical Practice": In the *Perspectives of a Century,* New York, Commonwealth Fund, 1945, p. 63. The ratio of physicians to population remains higher today in the United States than in Europe, but contrasts are not so extreme as a century ago. An American Medical Association committee reported in 1848 that this ratio was five times as great here as in France (Fishbein, M.: "History of American Medical Association," *J.A.M.A.,* 132: 852 (Dec. 7) 1946.

[15] Cobbett, W.: *The Rush-Light,* New York, Feb. 28, 1800.

and overcharging them in the process. The welfare of the public as well as self interest demanded that he be exposed.

It was gradually realized, however, that the scandal of medical quarrels was injuring the reputation of the profession. Even Rush, a born controversialist, sensed this in his last years. He then pleaded that physicians should cease to condemn one another just because of different theories of practice and urged that "the whole odium of the hostility of physicians" be ascribed to "their competition for business and money." [16]

Medical societies, fully aware of the frictions resulting from competition, sought to standardize principles of professional behavior. Percival's "medical ethics," adopted in London toward the end of the eighteenth century, was the basis of the code accepted by the American Medical Association at the time of its founding, and this English statement was also largely incorporated in the principles accepted by state and local societies.[17] These codes expressed certain general ideals and stated the duties of physicians to patients, to each other and to the public. They have since been criticized as providing "trade union rules" or "books of etiquette" rather than true ethics. Some critics object to the limitations set on criticisms of one physician by another, lest these shield the mediocre man at the expense of his patients. The codes may need overhauling today to fit them to modern conditions,[18] but any one who recalls the time when physicians did boast openly of their own

[16] Gross, S.: *Lives of Eminent American Physicians*, Philadelphia, Lindsay & Blakeston, 1861, p. 314; cited by Butterfield, L. H.: "Benjamin Rush: A Physician as Seen in His Letters," *Bull. Hist. Med.*, 20: 138 (July) 1946.

[17] Leake, C. D.: *Percival's Medical Ethics*, Baltimore, Williams & Wilkins Company, 1927, p. 33.

[18] That of the American Medical Association has been revised several times and is now being reconsidered again by the Judicial Council; Fishbein, M.: "History of American Medical Association," *J.A.M.A.*, 132: 783 (Nov. 30) 1946.

merits and of the inferiority of their rivals will recognize the
real service which these statements provided.

Even after medical societies had been organized there was
no little recrimination within the profession. In 1851, for
example, the therapeutic claims of a certain physician were
attacked on the floor of a state society. In retaliation the man
then published a pamphlet referring to the "meanness and
baseness" of the society's procedure, adding that the state
organization contained only "the pest boys and inexcusable
ignoramuses" of the profession. A member of the society,
writing to a colleague, began by inquiring: "Have you seen
the dirty pamphlet of Dr. X? . . . The more I reflect on this
man's attack on the state society the more angry I feel. . . .
After I read his account of pneumonia and his never having
lost a single case out of 179! I might have swallowed his
'obstetricy' (where did he get the word?) but I choked at his
pneumonia statistics. . . . I wish no controversy with such a
man . . . but I shrink from no responsibility." [19] One can see
from such correspondence that the officers of early medical
societies had their hands full in preserving professional harmony.

Long before ethical codes were adopted the early medical
societies had sought to deal with the strictly economic factor in
competition. They realized, apparently earlier than did business interests, that uncontrolled competition in an entirely
free market was not in the interests of competitors. Perhaps
the guild tradition in medicine had never permitted the
acceptance of a *laissez faire* philosophy so extreme as that
embraced by merchants. At any rate, a prime motive in the
founding of the pioneer state medical society (New Jersey,
1766) had been the standardization of fees. The fee bill issued
by that society listed charges of 25 cents and up for calls in

[19] Shryock, R. H.: "Selections from the Letters of Richard D. Arnold:
Medical Series, 1834–1875," *Bull. Johns Hopkins Hosp.*, 42: 156, 1928.

country practice, according to mileage, and such other items as $3.50 for deliveries. When it is recalled that annual tuition at Princeton was then only $4, these charges seem by no means low.[20]

Much the same comment may be made on the fee bills published by medical societies about seventy-five years later; that is, for the era just before the Civil War. Between 1835 and 1860, a fee of 50 cents or $1 was common for an office call at the physician's home in town practice, and rates were higher in the large cities.[21] These charges were at least the equivalent in purchasing power of $2 to $5 at the present time. Such comparisons are difficult to make for home calls, because the physician then charged in proportion to the distance traveled. The rural doctor also charged for medicines, so that it is hard to isolate the costs of professional services from those for drugs. Thus Dr. Tomlinson Fort of Milledgeville, Ga., included such items as the following in bills for 1841: [22]

> Visit, 4 miles in rain, and med............$ 7.00
> Visit, nocturnal, 4 miles................. 8.00
> Visit, 4 miles, $5.00 med., for gonorrhea.... 15.00

If one at least doubles these figures in order to estimate their purchasing power today, the fees seem relatively high.

Due allowance must be made here for certain variables. Dr. Fort's bills went to a planter who was probably wealthy and was perhaps charged accordingly. Bills sent to the rank and file may have been lower. Actual charges to most patients,

[20] Marsh, E. J.: "An Outline History of the Medical Society of New Jersey to 1903," *Proc. New Jersey Hist. Soc.,* 60: 5 (Jan.) 1942.

[21] Rosen, G.: "Fees and Fee Bills: Some Economic Aspects of Medical Practice in Nineteenth Century America," *Bull. Hist. Med.,* 1946, supp. 6, p. 11.

[22] Shryock, R. H.: "Medical Practice in the Old South," *South Atlantic Quart.,* 29: 173 (April) 1930.

moreover were some times less than those stated in the fee bills. There were complaints to this effect, for a published schedule was after all only a gentleman's agreement. But, keeping in mind all these factors, it seems likely that fees in general practice a century ago were little if any lower in real value than are current charges.

This is surprising when one recalls, first, how low the costs of medical education and equipment then were; and second, the common impression that rising professional costs have forced fees up since that time. Present protests against medical costs are not caused by higher fees in general practice but result rather from the many specialized services now required.

Had the average total cost of medical care been as high in 1846 as it is at present, it would have been quite impossible for the great majority of patients to have met it. The average, per capita real income then was less than half what it is today.[23] In other words, the ability to maintain present levels in medical costs—even as well as is now done—results from improvements in living standards all along the line.

Total medical costs were relatively low in 1846 because most persons were served simply by the family physician. Those in and near towns could reach pharmacists and dentists, and they occasionally resorted to consultants; but most rural folk, who then made up about 85 per cent of the population, received only bills for office or home calls from a single physician. Many of these charges, moreover, were not paid—a simple way of keeping down medical costs.

Difficulties in collecting fees inclined some physicians to accept so-called "contract practice." A physician would care for a family in return for a fixed payment in advance, perhaps for as little as $5 or $10 a year. There were then few opportunities for salaried positions, and contract work may have appealed to

[23] Martin, R. F.: National Income in the United States, 1799–1938; cited by Stern.[14]

practitioners in need of income. Similar procedures were sometimes followed in Europe, where they had had a long history.[24] The arrangement involved the prepayment principle for families only as a matter of individual agreement; whereas the insurance of entire groups, basic to current prepayment plans, was not introduced into American insurance until after 1910.[25] Just how extensive contract practice was in the United States before the Civil War is difficult to say, for one learns of it chiefly through objections voiced by professional leaders, who viewed the arrangement as demoralizing. It is doubtful if it was ever widely followed.

While on the subject of finances, one may well raise the old question: Why did the doctor's bill come last? The butcher, the baker, the candlestick-maker—all these must be paid promptly, but not the physician. Doctors themselves were none too meticulous about these matters, and many of them asked for settlement only at year's end. If not met then, the account was likely to go over another year, and so on. One of Dr. Fort's bills, noted previously, totaled $73.75. Under this was added the laconic statement: "8 yrs. int., 8%, $47.20."

The answer to the question just posed probably lies in the conflicting traditions of the profession. From the Middle Ages was inherited a semiclerical status—physicians should be more concerned with service than with profits. Hence arose the obligation to give freely to the poor, a generosity which was rarely expected of merchants. But modern capitalism had involved physicians in a competition for income which could not be ignored and which they tried to reconcile with the service ideal in ethical codes already mentioned.[26] The public,

[24] M. & S. *Reporter*, 1: 142, 1858. Letourneur, L. B. A.: "Rapports du médicin avec la société en général," thesis, Paris, no. 155, 1821, p. 26.

[25] Sickness benefits paid to members by lodges or mutual benefit societies, however, may be viewed as anticipating present group health insurance.

[26] Sigerist, H. E.: *Medicine and Human Welfare*, New Haven, Conn., Yale University Press, 1941, p. 116.

although it recognized medical charges as an obligation, tacitly assumed that these would not be pressed. Was not the physician the friend of the family, and was not this relationship above mercenary considerations? Professionally speaking, the practitioner thus lived a double life—half benefactor, half business man—with all the difficulties this entailed. The basic problem remains today, though it seems less acute under prevailing urban forms of practice.

Close personal relations between physicians and patients reflected both scientific and social conditions. Medical science, as will be noted later, then had small bearing on therapeutics. Hence few physicians felt it necessary to give much time to current scientific developments. They were, on the other hand, under constant pressure to meet the immediate needs of their neighbors. The established practitioner in the small urban or rural environment knew the lives of his patients and the affairs of the community. There was continuity in practice, for he had brought his patients into the world and seen their fathers out of it. Other things being equal, these circumstances were of real advantage in his work. The good family physician sensed environmental and personal factors in illness: he was his own medical social worker and authority on psychosomatic relationships. Mr. X would not be sick, his doctor would remark, if he could lift the mortgage on his farm. Mrs. Y's case needed what no one could give her—the return of her lost child. The physician would use either bread pills or bitter doses if these were indicated by personal factors. Most important on the psychic side was the influence of his own authority and personality. Here he was aided by the almost instinctive desire of patients to have faith in the man to whom they entrusted their lives.[27]

Although there was a growing tendency after 1830 to

[27] Pusey, W. A. : *A Doctor of the 1870's and '80's*, Springfield, Ill., Charles C Thomas, Publisher, 1932, p. 87.

distrust medical science in general, even the person who shared this feeling was apt to believe that his particular physician could always be of help.[28] Such faith, when misplaced, might have tragic consequences. Amid all the praise of the old family doctor it must be remembered that when incompetent he was of little use and may at times have done considerable harm. But faith in a competent man had its merits. The nice question, then as now, was how to distinguish between the able and the mediocre practitioner. Only in or near towns could there have been much range of choice, and in such locations the personal factor and sheer accident must have played major roles in the selection of family physicians. Hospital or medical school connections, often urged today as indications of professional merit, were then less significant or simply nonexistent. Graduates of certain schools seem to have had a superior reputation in special sections, as those of Harvard in New England, of Columbia and of Bellevue in New York and adjacent states, and of Pennsylvania and Jefferson in the Middle Atlantic area and the South. One authority at Yale suggested that patients, in considering a man as a prospective family physician, should engage him in conversation. If he spoke well on general matters the chances were that he was also intelligent in his practice. Beyond this there seems to have been little consideration of a problem which was so vital to the individual layman.[29]

Once having selected his physician, the American of the early nineteenth century was likely to place the greatest trust in him. Contemporary physicians might well envy the Dr. Watkins mentioned in the following note, in view of the

[28] See *North American Rev.*, 33: 368, 1831.
[29] Cf. Swackhamer, G.: *Choice and Change of Doctors,* New York Committee on Research in Medical Economics, 1939.

naive confidence displayed by his patient. The latter was Miss Virginia Randolph, a granddaughter of Thomas Jefferson and an intelligent and cultivated young woman. In a letter to her fiancé in 1822 she confided that: [30]

> We have had a rather sick family lately . . . and I am on Dr. Watkins' list. He has bled me twice, and prescribed a course of calomel which I am getting safely through . . . and I expect soon to be perfectly restored. You must not expect . . . that my health is worse than it frequently is, in summer, but Dr. Watkins wishes to make a permanent cure at once of all my complaints. . . . I have no doubt that his advice is most judicious.

The cynical reader will observe that it was the "course of calomel" rather than the illness which the patient was "getting safely through," and will no doubt marvel at Dr. Watkins' determination to cure *all* her difficulties *permanently* and *at once*. Yet Miss Randolph was probably none the worse for her faith in this case, and perhaps it sustained her in later and more serious "complaints."

The successful physician was then, as now, an overworked man. In the case of the city practitioner this was a matter of many patients—particularly if he were associated with a hospital. "The average of my private patients in the late summer and fall months," wrote a physician in 1849, "is generally between 30 and 40, and to get through with these . . . I am going the round from sunrise to 9 or 10 o'clock at night." In addition, he saw daily from 60 to 70 hospital patients. "The profession," he added on another occasion, "is one which certainly requires that a man should give up almost every social enjoyment and is therefore one which a person like myself who has so keen an enjoyment of such pleasures ought never to have chosen." [31]

[30] Randolph, V., to Nicholas Trist, Monticello, Va., July 26, 1822, in Trist Manuscripts, Library of Congress.
[31] Shryock,[19] Arnold to his daughter Ellen, Nov. 3, 1849, p. 170.

This does not mean that all physicians were denied social diversions, though clearly their evenings were not as free as those of other men, and they had little time for political activities or public affairs. Lawyers could run for legislature or Congress; physicians seldom had the time. In the large cities, however, prosperous physicians enjoyed the social life of medical clubs. One of the two original secretaries of the American Medical Association, en route to the organizing meeting in 1846, wrote as follows of professional hospitality in Philadelphia:

> This is a delightful House. . . . The assortment of wines, sherry, sauterne, champagne, and madeira was delicious. . . . After dinner we went to the Opera. . . . We were obliged to lose the third act, to go to Dr. Bell's Medical Club. The physicians here are very sociable amongst each other and meet three times a week at each other's houses. . . . We returned to the Opera and heard the third act and after that Dr. Clymer took me to the Club . . . I had an idea that they were all as stiff as if done up in buckram, but at this club, which is held at a large house in Walnut Street occupied solely by it, [there are] reading rooms below, card rooms and supper room on the second floor and billiard rooms on the third. I met Drs. Wm. Rush, Randolph, Biddle, Gerhard and Fox. . . . Without knowing it I played a game of five-dollar whist, but as soon as I was square I stopped playing.[32]

The country practitioner had no such opportunity for professional sociability, and such diversions as he had were those of the community at large. However, his lack of contact with colleagues was nothing like the deprivation that this seems today in isolated areas. The nature of practice was so simple that there seemed little technical need for a hospital or for professional discussions. Deliveries were made at home,

[32] Shryock,[19] Arnold to his wife, April 13, 1846, p. 166.

and the kitchen table still seemed adequate for emergency surgical procedures. Incidentally, the introduction of anesthesia in the late 'forties aided surgical practice in country homes as well as in city hospitals.

The rural physician handled all phases of practice, including pharmacy and dentistry. While he saw fewer patients than did his urban colleague, he was kept just as busy by long hours spent on the road. It is not easy to picture this old routine, though much has been written about "the horse and buggy doctor." As a matter of fact, the buggy was not the only means of transportation. The physician often rode an old mare equipped with saddlebags which contained drugs and a surgical kit. He was on the road so much of the time that he could have no regular office hours: patients must take their chances on finding him at home. When a railroad reached a community, the physician would use that if possible, sometimes being extended the doubtful privilege of riding the freight cars. Occasionally he even sallied forth on a "railroad tricycle," similar to the later handcar.[33] These devices, like runaway horses or modern automobiles, had their own peculiar risks.

One form of practice was peculiar to the days before the Civil War. This was the care of slaves. On southern farms of moderate size practice was usually in the hands of the mistress or of overseers, who were guided by tradition and by family medical manuals. Dr. Samuel Cartwright referred in 1850 to "the practice among 3 millions of people [Negroes] that the overseers have mostly got." [34] Even slaves themselves occasionally acquired a reputation as folk practitioners.

It was argued in defense of slavery that it gave the master a

[33] Pusey,[27] p. 39. Hertzler, A. E.: *The Horse and Buggy Doctor*, New York, Harper & Brothers, 1938, p. 61.

[34] Cited by Fenner, E. D.: *Southern Medical Reports*, New Orleans, B. M. Norman, D. Davies & Son, 1850–1851, vol. 2, p. 423.

financial interest in preserving the health of his "people," and this was doubtless true in the case of the more enlightened and prosperous planters. Such men would hire Irish laborers rather than put their slaves into dangerous work. If a slave died, there was a loss of several hundred dollars; if an Irishman perished, there was just one less Irishman in the world! [35]

Wealthy planters would regularly employ a prominent local physician to look after their plantations. This gave slaves as good care as was then available and provided them with a rough equivalent of modern health insurance. There were certain legal aspects here which were peculiar to slavery. In cases which required surgical intervention, for example, the master's permission rather than that of the patient was required. (In one curious instance the great gynecologist Marion Sims could not secure such permission and actually purchased a patient in order to operate on her.[36]) After emancipation most of this service was lost, and the rural southern Negro now receives less medical care than do members of any other large element in the population.

Implicit in all that has been said is the fact that nearly all physicians in 1846 were general practitioners. Certain persons became especially interested in surgery, but they seldom abandoned general practice entirely. This combination of the physician and surgeon in one practitioner came down from a time of primitive colonial conditions, when differentiation would have been impractical. As a result surgery always maintained equal prestige with internal medicine, in contrast to the professional and social distinctions which had been traditional in Britain.

It is usually assumed that specialization was lacking at this time simply because there was not enough knowledge to

[35] Phillips, U. B.: *Life and Labor in the Old South*, Boston, Little, Brown & Co., 1929, p. 186.
[36] Shryock,[22] p. 172.

justify it. This was indeed one factor in the situation. But there was another basic explanation. Prior to about 1830 American physicians did not usually think in terms of a localized pathologic process or of specific diseases. Speculative pathologies had dominated medical thought up to that time. All forms of illness were ascribed to one or two generalized conditions, such as impurities of the blood or the existence of excessive tension or laxity in the nervous and vascular systems. These were appealing theories, since they solved all pathologic problems at once and also opened up a royal road in therapeutics. If all illness was due, as Benjamin Rush claimed, to excessive tension in the blood vessels, then all patients could be cured by bleeding to relieve that tension. Any one could see that if the patient was bled long enough he would relax— sooner or later! Hence the physician should put no faith in the healing powers of nature but rather should interfere with nature as promptly as possible.

As long as all forms of illness were viewed as expressing a single, underlying condition, there was no occasion for specialization in practice. Every physician considered that he had the remedy that was "good for what ailed you," since by definition the same thing ailed every one. Incidentally, there was also no use for major surgical operations, for one could hardly operate on the blood or on a vague condition common to the whole vascular system.[37] Hence surgical practice remained largely a matter of fractures, amputations and other superficial emergencies, and here again there was little need for specialization.

Only when a localized, structural basis for pathology replaced the speculative systems was specialization made possible. When specific diseases were identified by correlating lesions with symptoms, the possibility of treatment by remov-

[37] Sigerist, H. E.: "Surgery at the Time of the Introduction of Antisepsis," *J. Missouri M. A.*, 32: 169, 1935.

ing these lesions became obvious. Surgery was therefore beginning, by 1840, to move from the periphery toward the center of medical practice. And there was now some reason for specializing, in other fields than surgical practice, in work on a particular part or system.[38] But these new points of view, imported from Paris by returning American students after 1820, percolated slowly into average practice. Not until after the Civil War did specialization really get under way, even in the cities.[39] There was strong opposition at first, partly because of the fear that it would injure the interests of both patient and practitioner,[40] partly because in the earlier day only quacks had claimed to specialize. Dr. S. Weir Mitchell could recall the time in Philadelphia when to specialize meant to be professionally ostracized.[41]

The French school of 1800–50 was as critical of the traditional therapeutics as it was of the older pathologies. Since it identified diseases by symptoms as well as by lesions found at autopsy, it developed methods for improving clinical observation. The stethoscope and clinical statistics are cases in point. But the use of the latter showed the ineffectiveness of bleeding, purging and the old drugs. Hence French clinicians gradually lost interest in therapeutics. How could there be an intelligent search for the causes and cures of diseases until the diseases themselves had first been found?

Medical research thereupon become nihilistic; it was focused on diagnosis rather than on treatments. The latter were

[38] Rosen, G.: *The Specialization of Medicine,* New York, Froben Press, 1944, p. 15.

[39] The gradual transition from general practice to specialization in surgery in a small city about 1880 is described in Wheeler, J. B.: *Memoirs of a Small-Town Surgeon,* New York, Garden City Publishing Company, 1935, p. 176.

[40] Ware, J.: "Success in the Medical Profession," Introductory Lecture, Massachusetts Medical College, Boston, D. Clapp, 1851, p. 9.

[41] Mitchell, S. W.: "The History of Instrumental Precision in Medicine," *Univ. M. Mag.,* 4: 1, 1891.

viewed as useless in most cases. Oliver Wendell Holmes, on his return from Paris, informed the American people that if most of the medicines used here were thrown into the sea it would be all the better for mankind and all the worse for the fishes! [42] What was needed, he felt, was less medical interference and a revived confidence in the healing powers of nature. This critical view affected average practice only after a long interval; indeed, Osler was still preaching it in the first edition of his textbook near the close of the century.[43]

It is true that by the 'fifties some younger physicians indoctrinated by French-trained professors were becoming less inclined to bleed and purge, less given to excessive medication. But most practitioners clung to traditional forms of treatment. Some of the older men, even those who taught in the better schools, were still defending venesection in the 'seventies.[44] This half century lag in bringing practice into harmony with research is an interesting phenomenon which has never been adequately studied.

In reaction to such professional conservatism, popular opposition developed against heroic treatments. Such was the protest against calomel (mild mercurous chloride), for example, that a large and thriving medical sect—the Thomsonian or "Botanic System"—based its appeal on the condemnation of all mineral or metallic remedies that had come into use since the days of Paracelsus. Echoes of its propaganda survive today in the advertisements of secret remedies that "contain only vegetable compounds."

Popular distrust of medical treatments was based, by 1840,

---

[42] Holmes, O. W.: *Currents and Counter-Currents in Medical Science,* Boston, Ticknor & Fields, 1861, p. 39.

[43] By that time such nihilism was almost out of date, for pharmacology and bacteriology already held real promise for both prevention and cure.

[44] I.e., as a general procedure in many forms of illness. See, e.g., Littell, S.: "Memoir of George B. Wood," *Trans. Coll. Physicians, Philadelphia,* 5: XXV, 1881. Shryock,[1] p. 135.

on more than a dislike of unpleasant or dangerous remedies. By this time physical science was making such headway that all could appreciate it. But where were the *medical* equivalents of the steam engine or the telegraph? Medicine seemed to have fallen behind the other sciences: indeed, the leading professors of medicine now admitted that their science was of little utility. Perhaps the old medical "systems," with their speculative pathologies, were really more valuable. They had at least promised cures. So encouraged, various theorists revived the doctrine that there was one cause and therefore one cure of disease. Thus Hahnemann reduced most pathologic conditions to the itch and most treatments to the "like cures like" theory and the high dilution formulas, somewhat as Dr. Still would later reduce all pathologic processes to spinal conditions and all therapeutic practice to spinal manipulations.

Regular medicine, which had accepted such oversimplifications in Rush's day, was now more critical and would have none of them. Homeopaths and Thomsonians thereupon became the modern medical sects. They founded their own schools and journals and so contributed to the confusion in education and licensing which has previously been mentioned.[45] On the other hand, the sects probably did more than did French nihilism to create a salutary demand for milder treatments.

The more credulous or nervous folk also flocked to a whole series of minor cults which promised sure and pleasant cures. Nearly every conceivable type of humbug preyed on the people—hydropathy, chronothermalism, mesmerism, herb doctors, faith doctors, indianopathists and what you will!

[45] Some forty Thomsonian journals were published in the United States between 1825 and 1850. For bibliography of the sects, Shryock, R. H.: "Public Relations of the Medical Profession in Great Britain and United States," *Ann. M. Hist.*, 2: 308, 1930 [notes 41–44].

Meanwhile national advertising in newspapers was originated by the manufacturers of secret remedies, and more money was spent for nostrums than for prescriptions. When regular physicians protested, they were viewed merely as opposing competitors. Was not this a free country, and did not every American have an inalienable right to life, liberty, and quackery? A writer in one of the journals of opinion suggested that "the public will act as an umpire" between the regulars and the sectarians, and reach its decision "after a careful perusal of the undertaker's bills." [46]

It is to be recalled that this was an age of social ferment and reform, the day of the great temperance, antislavery, and women's right movements as well as of minor utopian aspirations. "We learn from the papers," observed Dr. William Alcott in 1835, "that the American Seventh Commandment Society, the New York Female Benevolent Society, the New York Ladies' Moral Reform Society, and the Anti-Tobacco Society held their annual meetings at New York about the middle of May, and that some of these meetings were interesting." [47] In such an atmosphere it was natural that a utopian health cult should arise, advising all to maintain health by staying away from the physicians and by cultivating personal hygiene. Their views represented the logical extreme of the "trust nature" philosophy, which was preached in more moderate form by physicians who had been influenced by French nihilism. Sylvester Graham, the leader of the cult, preached during the 'forties the virtues of bathing, of exercise and of a whole-wheat diet. In his spare time he originated an interesting literary tradition later known by the phrase "What a Young Man Should Know." His antimedical doctrine was spread by "Ladies Physiological Reform Societies," and he is

[46] "The Medical Controversy," *United States Democratic Rev.*, 35: 263, 1855.
[47] *Boston Moral Reformer*, 1: 225, 1835.

unconsciously recalled to this day in the terms "Graham bread" and "Graham crackers." [48]

The appeal for personal hygiene had some merit at a time when the Saturday night bath was a real victory for sweetness and light. But more significant was the public hygiene of the period. About the end of the eighteenth century, the medieval doctrine of contagion in epidemics was partially replaced by a revival of the classic "airs and waters" hypothesis. If epidemics originated in the local contamination of air and water, then quarantines were of little use. "Noxious Miasms" could be eliminated only by cleanups, by sanitary reform. Philadelphia led the way, after its bitter experiences with yellow fever, in constructing one of the first steam-powered water works in the country (1802) and by other municipal improvements. Bitter controversy continued, however, over whether certain diseases were spread by miasms or by contagion.

Quite naturally, as epidemic diseases were more clearly identified, distinct causal factors were sought in terms of one of these theories or the other. Specific pathology led in turn to a search for specific etiology. Those who held to miasms tried to find poisons in the air peculiar to given diseases, while those who accepted contagion turned to the old theory that animalcules or micro-organisms might convey specific infections. Such American physicians as Daniel Drake of Cincinnati, J. C. Nott of Mobile, Ala., and J. K. Mitchell of Philadelphia wrote during the 1840's in support of the animalcular hypothesis.[49] Their views, based on an intelligent interpretation of epidemiologic data, represented more than mere speculation. But they failed to verify their theories by laboratory studies. Hence the pioneer work in parasitology and medical bacteri-

[48] See Chapter V.
[49] Allen, P., "Etiological Theory in America Prior to the Civil War," *J. Hist. Med. & Allied Sc.*, 2:489–520, 1947.

ology between 1840 and 1870 was left largely to Europeans.

The failure of Americans to contribute much to medical science prior to the present century may be explained by a number of factors.[50] Notable was the indifference of a commercially-minded people to research that promised no immediate utility. Why should any one encourage studies in pathology or in physiology, if these were of no help to patients? Professional prestige here was acquired rather through a fashionable practice, which presumably aided the sick and at the same time bore the hallmark of financial success. Such a practice left small time for original investigations.[51]

It is true that a few physicians also acquired reputations through professorships and consulting practices, but this was by no means the same thing as research. These men edited European works, "putting British portraits of disease in American frames," and occasionally compiled textbooks of their own; but it is remarkable how infrequently even the famous professors made any systematic investigations. A committee of the American Medical Association reported in 1850 that only two "experimental memoirs" of any importance had appeared during the preceding year—one on poisons and one on the nervous system of the alligator.[52]

While the American public was relatively indifferent to pure science, it was much concerned with applied science. Hence arose all the debate about medical practice and the search for immediate cures. Most pressing in the public mind was the fear of epidemics. Outbreaks of yellow fever had inspired the beginnings of sanitary reform by 1800, but it was

[50] Shryock, R. H.: *American Medical Research: Past and Present,* New York, Commonwealth Fund, 1947.

[51] See the contemporary protest against this situation in Jackson, S.: *Address to the Medical Graduates of the University of Pennsylvania,* Philadelphia, T. K. & P. G. Collins, 1840, p. 15.

[52] Fishbein, M.: "History of American Medical Association," *J.A.M.A.,* 132: 920 (Dec. 14) 1946.

the terrifying specter of cholera which during the 'thirties and again in the 'fifties aroused a real demand for protection. Meanwhile, municipal authorities were disturbed by the rising death rates of various communicable diseases and learned with interest of similar concern abroad. Since sanitation seemed as much a matter for engineers and statisticians as for physicians, laymen at first assumed leadership in the public health movement. Thus Lemuel Shattuck, onetime teacher, submitted an excellent plan for a state department of health in Massachusetts (1850), which was in part the basis for the state board eventually set up there in 1869.

A few socially minded physicians realized, however, that public health programs needed medical as well as mathematical guidance. At the start of its career the American Medical Association appointed a committee on public hygiene, which submitted valuable reports on the sanitary—or rather, unsanitary—condition of American cities and called for remedial legislation.

Soon after these reports had been made, one of the leaders of the Northern Medical Association took the center of the national stage. It happened that an international sanitary conference was called in Paris in 1855 in order to discuss cooperation in quarantine legislation. This suggested to Dr. Wilson Jewell, of the Philadelphia Board of Health, that state quarantine laws were just as diverse in the United States as were national statutes in Europe and that Americans faced the same need for coordination. He therefore persuaded his board to call a national sanitary convention, which met in Philadelphia in 1857. Subsequent meetings were held, during the ensuing three years, in Baltimore, New York, and Boston. Municipal officials and socially minded physicians joined in discussions of quarantines, sanitary regulations, and the need for pure food and drug laws. This principle of bringing laymen and physicians together for the promotion of health programs was later to be employed effectively by such voluntary organizations as the National Tuberculosis Association.

Jewell was the leading spirit in these first national sanitary conventions. That of 1860 planned to transform the meetings into a permanent national health association, but the session of 1861 was unfortunately prevented by the Civil War.[53] A national body was not actually formed until the American Public Health Association came into being in 1872. It would be interesting if more could be learned about Dr. Jewell, both in relation to his leadership in health reform and to his professional career in Philadelphia. It is ironic that a leader who felt he had inaugurated "a new era in the domain of American Science"[54] has been so largely forgotten in the annals of public health.

This brings me back to my starting point, the advent of this Association, for Jewell was one of its founders.[55] Evidently he was concerned with the problems of private practice as well as with those of public hygiene. Not all aspects of such practice have been considered here, but enough has been said to suggest that the physician of a century ago faced some problems that were peculiar to his time and others which persist today. The better physicians of 1846 would be proud of the present status of medical science and of the medical guild. Indeed they would be amazed by it all. The physician of today also should take a little pride in them, for they labored long under difficult circumstances to advance the interests of their patients and of their profession.

[53] On Jewell's leadership, see his letter to Dr. J. H. Griscom, in the Proceedings of the Third National Quarantine and Sanitary Convention, New York, 1859, pp. 3 ff. Plans for a permanent national association are noted in *Proceedings and Debates*, Fourth National Quarantine and Sanitary Convention, Boston, 1860, p. 8.

[54] Jewell's words at the first meeting in Philadelphia.

[55] A centennial history of the Association has been prepared by its president, Dr. Maurice Jacobs.

IX

Women in American Medicine *

It is auspicious that the section on Medical History of the College of Physicians should associate itself with the history of women in American medicine, as the subject for this lecture in the series provided for by the late Dr. Kate C. Hurd-Mead. Much of the literature concerning the entrance of women into the medical profession has dealt with this as a new or experimental movement. Hence it comes almost as a shock to realize that it is now a full century since the founding of the Woman's Medical College of Pennsylvania. This, the earliest and now the only such school in the western world, may well serve as a symbol of the entire story. It is already, as things go in this country, a venerable institution; and I feel honored by this opportunity to salute it on the occasion of its centenary.

The story of women in American medicine involves chapters in the history of medicine, of women, and of American society; no one of which is intelligible save in relation to the others. To do this full justice, one should possess many qualifications; but perhaps you will be tolerant for the moment of the limited perspective of the historian. I shall not attempt to trace the actual records of individuals and institutions, since these have already been treated by Dr. Hurd-Mead and by

* Reprinted from *Journal of the American Medical Women's Association,* Vol. 5, No. 9, September, 1950—by permission.

other able medical women.[1] It would seem more pertinent to analyze topically certain of the trends and issues of the last hundred years. With this in mind, the subject can be resolved into a discussion, first, of the factors which originally favored women in medicine; second, of those which opposed them; third, of the major trends; and, fourth, of the outcomes. Much of this must be made brief, although the story is so human that there is a constant temptation to digress or to indulge in details.

Consider, first, the factors which favored the entrance of women into medicine. American society a century ago was in a state of "transition." For centuries women had been almost completely subordinated to men under both common and statute law. This situation, whatever its hidden implications, elicited little open protest from women in such a simple, agrarian society as obtained in this country until after 1800. Colonial women lived on the farms, and their sphere was of necessity the home. Thereafter, however, the industrial revolution began to attract both sexes into the cities—where poor women made the first break with the home by entering the mills. There were also numbers of middle-class women who became teachers; while others found themselves endowed with sufficient property and leisure to become concerned about their own interests. Meantime, the so-called enlightenment of the later 1700's had encouraged a belief in the perfectibility of society by a resort to reason rather than by mere dependence on tradition or authority. This faith in "progress" produced a veritable rush of social reform which reached its high point during the 1840's and 1850's.

By this time, the calm and rational appeals of the enlight-

[1] Marshall, C., "The Woman's Medical College of Pennsylvania: a History," *Virginia M. Semi-Monthly,* Jan. 27, '99.

Hurd-Mead, K. C., *Medical Women of America,* New York, Froben, 1933.

Selmon, B. L., Series of papers in *M. Women's J.,* 1945–1949.

enment had been suffused with the emotion of a more romantic age and even took on something of an evangelical enthusiasm. We all recall, as examples, the temperance and anti-slavery crusades; but we overlook the many less well-known movements.

One of these reform drives was the women's rights movement, made feasible by the economic changes mentioned but consciously directed by leaders, journals, and societies. "Ladies' magazines," demanding equal rights, had appeared in Philadelphia as early as the 1790's; and the movement was in full swing when its first convention was held in 1848. It hardly need be added that equal educational opportunities and the right to enter the professions were among the demands of the militant minority which aided this cause. The desire of a few women to enter medicine and the support given them can only be understood against this larger background.

Feminists at large saw in the admittance of women to medicine a dramatic test case for their whole movement, and encouraged it at every opportunity. Thus Sarah Josepha Hale, editor of *Godey's Ladies Book,* remarked tartly in 1852: "Talk about this [medicine] being the appropriate sphere for man, and his alone! With tenfold more plausibility and reason, we say it is the appropriate sphere for woman, and hers alone." [2] In any case, the feminists held, women had the same rights as did men to enter a profession of their choice.

The desire for equal rights was not the only influence which impinged upon women at this juncture. Another of the now forgotten crusades was that for reform in personal hygiene. This was led in the 1840's by one Sylvester Graham. Besides urging dietary improvements, Graham was concerned about sex hygiene and advocated dress reform and physical exercise for women. His feminine audiences responded by

[2] Quoted in Woody, T., *History of Women's Education in the United States,* Lancaster, Pa., Science Press, 1929, II, 344.

organizing "Ladies Physiological Reform Societies," and daring women—notably, Paulina Wright—began to lecture to them on anatomy and physiology. This teaching of both sex and general hygiene called for medically trained women as instructors, and many of the first women who entered medicine had this objective clearly in mind. At first they lectured to voluntary groups, as had Paulina Wright; later they would be appointed to advise or direct women in schools and other institutions.

The desire to provide women for such instruction was related to a broader demand for practitioners of their sex in obstetrics and gynecology. Those seeking equal professional rights in principle, recalled indignantly that the practice of midwifery had long been "a woman's sphere." But male physicians had gradually taken this practice away from the midwives after 1780, among the native white population, in the name of more expert service. This change did not occur without some protest, which perhaps never entirely disappeared; but a more vocal reaction against it arose during the 1840's. It was proclaimed in no uncertain terms that attendance by men in obstetric cases was offensive to modesty, and that, partly for that reason, the medical results were also unfortunate. As an added argument, it was claimed that once a mother's modesty was gone, chastity would follow it.[3]

We need not linger over this picture of a universal corruption of the American home, but one thing should be pointed out. It was in this early Victorian period that middle-class, Anglo-Saxon prudery was carried to the most extreme lengths. When Paulina Wright was so brazen as to discuss anatomy before the ladies, many of them had recourse to smelling salts and there were frequent faintings. Now just to

[3] Gregory, S., *Man-Midwifery Exposed and Corrected,* Boston, George Gregory, 1848, pp. 18 ff. See also his *Letters to Ladies in Favor of Female Physicians,* New York, Fowler and Wells, 1850.

the extent that this excessive delicacy was cultivated in the "genteel female," she suffered when suddenly exposed to male practitioners. There is abundant evidence that many women avoided medical attention for serious conditions or concealed much from such doctors as they did consult, because of this embarrassment. While some physicians deplored this situation,[4] others actually gloried in it as evidence of the high moral tone of their generation.[5]

It is most puzzling, in view of the growing prudishness of Anglo-Saxon society between 1800 and 1850, that women were ever persuaded to abandon midwives. Logically, one would have expected the English and Americans to cling to them longer than did realistic Latin peoples; but actually the reverse was true. The most prudish gave up the services of their own sex most readily.

Whatever the explanation of this paradox in our social history, one way in which to meet the difficulties of the 1840's was to revive the waning service of midwives. Since the original objection to them had been their ignorance, why not undertake their serious training? Dr. Shippen had attempted this when he gave the first American lectures on obstetrics. Midwives trained under Shippen probably had as good a course as was then available in this country, and were probably still practicing as late as 1800. The following advertisement appeared in the *Delaware Gazette* of October 31, 1789:

> Grace Mulligan takes this opportunity to inform the public that she has been solicited to come to Wilmington to practice Midwifery; she has had the advantage of the instructions . . . of Dr. Shippen in Philadelphia better

[4] Shryock, R. H., editor, *The Arnold Letters*, Trinity College Historical Papers, Duke University Press, 1929, XVIII, p. 18.

[5] Meigs, C. D., *Females and Their Diseases*, Philadelphia, Lea and Blanchard, 1848. (Dr. Meigs took this view, though he hoped something could be done to decrease embarrassment.)

than a year, and comes recommended by him in the most flattering terms.

Schools for midwives were also set up in most European countries. One wonders, in passing, why such schools did not develop here and in England as in Continental Europe, and whether routine might not have been the better for it if this had been the American outcome. Be that as it may, the attempt to revive their training was made by Dr. Samuel Gregory of Boston, who established there a college for midwives in 1848. In a series of exchanges with local medical bodies, he publicized the need for women in the service of their own sex.[3] This same need was voiced by the early women's medical schools and hospitals, which therefore emphasized the practice of obstetrics and gynecology. Women who desired full medical training, however, could not well support Gregory's program for the revival of midwifery. On this point they were of necessity aligned with other physicians, who urged a complete medical education for all who practiced obstetrics. Nevertheless, the abortive attempt to bring back the midwives probably aided women doctors by publicizing the sex issue in medical practice.

A minor factor favoring the entrance of women into medicine, was the low state of practice during the mid-nineteenth century. This was the era of proprietary schools, when almost anyone could be licensed after two terms of lectures, and the profession must have been full of mediocre men or worse. One senses a hope, indeed a determination, among early women leaders to improve this situation wherever possible.

The very opposition which women encountered from the profession, moreover, was in one sense a blessing in disguise, for it placed women upon their mettle. Now what was the nature of this opposition? Basically, of course, it was a man's world and men intended to keep it that way. Or one should say, rather, that *most* of them had this intention; for at every point—as in the feminist movement as a whole—there were individual men who supported the cause. These leaders and some able men who have served on the staff of the Woman's Medical College here should receive due recognition. Probably the great majority of men and a considerable proportion of women, however, opposed the presence of the so-called "weaker sex" in medicine. Fortunately, however, there was sufficient liberalism in the air to make even conservative doctors feel that explanations of this attitude were necessary.

The subserviency of women in general, and their exclusion from professions in particular, were first of all justified by traditional opinions anent differences between the sexes. Lacking our present life expectancy figures, men then cherished the illusion that females were the weaker sex and were therefore less able to stand the strain of practice. But it was upon the supposed mental differences that the opposition really concentrated. Women were said to be modest, dependent, retiring; they were lacking in courage and originality. They were, by nature, fitted for the care of the home, but disqualified for activities in more worldly spheres. In thus ascribing temperamental differences to innate nature, all the influences of the surrounding culture were ignored. Recall that this was a romantic and sentimental age, when every effort was made to render women as distinctively feminine as possible. These efforts were made, of course, in the name of "sweetness and light." Women were formed of finer and more sensitive stuff than men: it was everyone's wish to protect them from the harsher realities.

Let me quote just one of the contemporary sentimental tributes to women, in which I think you will detect an undertone of condescension in the very midst of flowery tributes. "The great administrative faculties," observed a distinguished physician, "are not found in women":

> The Forum is no theater for her silvery voice. She discerns not the course of the planets. Orion with his belt, and Arcturus with his suns are naught to her but pretty baubles set up in the sky. She composes no *Iliad,* no *Aeneid.* . . . Such is not woman's province, nature, power, or mission. She reigns in the heart. . . . Home is her place, except when, like the star of day, she deigns to issue forth to the world, to exhibit her beauty and her grace . . . and then she goes back to her home, like as the sun sinks in the west, and the memory of her presence is like a bright departed day.

All this, believe it or not, appeared in a textbook on obstetrics of 1848. At a time when phrenology was still taken seriously, this author concluded with the telling observation that: "She has a head almost too small for intellect but just big enough for love."

Medical women, in the face of such comments, usually kept silent or replied with restraint. But they were sorely tried by those of their own sex who seemed willing to accept these indictments, and, as it were, to live up to them. In the first Annual Announcement of the Woman's Medical College of Pennsylvania, it was observed that girls themselves had often been deterred from an interest in medicine by the

> absurd arguments of those [women], the exercise of whose mental abilities seldom reach beyond the decorations of the boudoir and toilet, and we find that those who have been deaf to such idle protestations of delicate imbecility, have shed luster on Literature and Science. . . .

Those who viewed women as unfitted for professional work naturally concluded that any who attempted it could do so only by imitating the men. Dr. Alfred Stillé, in his presidential address before the American Medical Association in 1871, declared that:

> Certain women seek to rival men in manly sports . . . and the strong-minded ape them in all things, even in dress. In doing so, they may command a sort of admiration such as all monstrous productions inspire, especially when they tend towards a higher type than their own.[6]

Actually, of course, any tendency to imitate male colleagues elicited ridicule rather than admiration, a ridicule which appealed to the common distaste for mannish women and for effeminate men. As late as 1910, there was a popular impression that medical women could be recognized on the streets by dress and bearing.

There is no telling just how much ridicule of this sort handicapped women physicians. They were at a disadvantage here, because in a profession where all the norms had been set by men some imitation was inevitable. The obstacles facing women, moreover, inspired a challenge only in those who were unusually resolute and determined. Since these qualities were among those usually ascribed to males, it followed almost by definition that medical women would be popularly viewed as mannish in temperament. When psychologists worked out tests for masculinity and femininity, by the 1930's, they reported that women holding the M.D. or Ph.D. degree rated high in masculinity. But one wonders just what such scales, based on general impressions of sex differences, really mean.[7] Moreover, women were almost goaded into some impersonation of men by the very arguments used against them. Informed that their sex was too delicate to undertake medical

---

[6] Transactions of the American Medical Assn., 1871, XXII, p. 75 ff. Fishbein, M., *History of the American Medical Association*, Philadelphia, W. B. Saunders Company, 1947, p. 90.

[7] Terman, L. M., and Miles, C. C., *Sex and Personality*, New York, McGraw-Hill Company, 1936, pp. 182, 578.

pursuits, they had to prove that they were really tough and could "take it." But this only brought down again upon them the ridicule of mannishness. They could not win either way.

Perhaps, too, the women were at a disadvantage in denying the super-delicacy of their sex by the fact that they themselves had resorted to this notion in connection with obstetrics. In this field, they were great believers in feminine delicacy, but they denied that this quality need be taken seriously when it came to their own presence in medical schools. If this was inconsistent, it was no more so than the logic of the conservatives who simply reversed the reasoning. For the latter, feminine modesty was too fine a thing to be sacrificed for medical training; but when it came to obstetrical practice, it appeared that modesty could be completely ignored.

In medicine, as in other professions, women were obviously handicapped by social inertia. The fact that all American physicians had hitherto been men made the very thought of a "doctress" seem absurd to many persons. When the first "females" entered a medical class, they must have appeared more bizarre than would today the appearance of a single male at Vassar. It was easy to believe that such women were queer persons. It is not surprising that people made fun of them, and that a little of this found its way into print. In 1874, for example, a work by one Max Adeler portrayed a professor at the Woman's Medical College in Philadelphia. This lady was such an enthusiast for science that she would administer chloroform to her husband during his afternoon naps, and then "demonstrate" him to a class disguised as a sewing circle. On the particular occasion described, however, the instruction could not be carried very far because, as the professor observed: ". . . Mr. Magruder's system was somewhat debilitated [by] . . . an overdose of chlorate of potash which she had administered in his coffee . . . for the purpose of testing the strength of the drug." [8]

It may be that the inclination to make fun of a "doctress" was not equally shared on all social levels. The genteel classes, always sensitive about the proprieties, were probably most startled by this new phenomenon. On the other hand, the early experience of the women's hospitals suggests that poor women resorted to them with little hesitation.[9] Perhaps they cared less about appearances and respectability. Or, if immigrants, they may have welcomed "the doctoring ladies" because they had already been accustomed to the services of midwives.

There was no little suspicion that doctors opposed medical women for fear of economic competition, the usual motive for suppressing a minority element. Occasionally, this matter came out into the open, as when an article in the Boston Medical Journal noted as early as 1853 that competition was becoming serious; women were already cutting in on the profits in obstetric cases.[10] In the same city Dr. Gregory, who suffered from no inhibitions, accused the doctors of desiring a male monopoly of the market. In so far as fear of competition promoted all sorts of rationalizations, it was unfortunate for women that the medical profession was over-supplied during the last half of the nineteenth century. The ratio of doctors to population was far higher here than in Europe, and competition within the profession was already keen when women began to enter it. Had there been a dearth of practitioners, opposition to the latter would doubtless have been less, as is

[8] Adeler, M., *Out of the Hurly-Burly*, Philadelphia, George Maclean, 1874, pp. 71 ff.

[9] Blackwell, Emily, "New York Infirmary for Women and Children," *Trans. Woman's Medical College of Pennsylvania Alumnae*, Philadelphia, 1900, p. 76–80.

[10] *Boston M. J.*, 48: 66, 1853.

suggested by the somewhat contrasting experience in Russia, when women first entered the medical schools there in the 1870's. After the first medical school for women was opened in St. Petersburg (1872), nearly 700 women took medical degrees there within the one decade between 1878 and 1888.[11]

Certain other characteristics of the profession besides overcrowding operated to the disadvantage of women. Low-grade medical schools had attracted low-grade students, and the latter were viewed even in the public press as an uncouth and "licentious" lot.[12] This explains the extraordinary boorishness displayed by some student groups toward the first women who attended hospital clinics—one of the most trying experiences with which the latter had to contend. In contrast, Mary Putnam met with only the most gentlemanly consideration from fellow students at Paris in the early 1870's.

The division of the medical profession between the regulars and the sects also caused some confusion among medical women. Homeopathy, eclecticism, and other groups were then a real threat to the "allopaths," and feeling was bitter.[13] The sects, struggling for existence, were more open-minded about accepting women. An eclectic school at Rochester admitted them as early as 1849, at about the same time that Elizabeth Blackwell received from the Geneva Medical College the first "regular" medical degree granted to a woman in this country. Other irregular colleges welcomed both sexes during the 1850's and 1860's. Anxious to avoid any appearance of sectarianism, however, the Woman's Medical College of Pennsylvania cleared its original faculty of irregulars, and several other women's schools followed suit. Women were

[11] Kasakovitch, H., *Trans. Woman's Medical College of Pennsylvania Alumnae*, Philadelphia, 1900, pp. 61–66.

[12] Philadelphia City *Item*, November 6, 1858, for example.

[13] Shryock, R. H., "Quackery and Sectarianism in American Medicine," *The Scalpel of Alpha Epsilon Delta*, May, '49.

thus divided between the orthodox and the heretics, and weakened accordingly. A national organization of women homeopaths was formed in 1904, and an osteopathic group in 1914, before the regular Medical Women's National Association, now the American Medical Women's Association, was founded in 1915.

A final obstacle to the full admission of women into medicine was presented by the multiple lines of conservative defense. If one were scaled, the opposition re-formed in the rear. If women could get into schools, the hospitals were still closed; and if the latter were finally opened, internships and residencies were still denied them. When "doctoring ladies" appeared, physicians refused to consult with them and prevented their entrance into medical societies. In 1870 the Montgomery County Society opened its portals, and in 1876 the American Medical Association seated a delegate from Illinois.[14] But other societies held out longer, and, meantime, women encountered long delays in securing appointments to hospital staffs. After World War I, however, exclusive national bodies and specialist societies displayed less resistance; by 1932, for example, sixty-nine women were members of the College of Surgeons.[15] In 1930, Dr. Catharine Macfarlane became a member of the College of Physicians of Philadelphia, the oldest medical academy in the country; and Dr. Margaret Sturgis and several other women have since been honored in the same manner. But it is clear, throughout the story, that women had to penetrate defense in depth.

From the start, women were divided among themselves as to the merits of separate schools. The latter were founded only after the established colleges had refused to accept "female"

[14] Fishbein, M., *History of the American Medical Association,* Philadelphia, W. B. Saunders Company, 1947, pp. 85, 91.
[15] Hurd-Mead, K. C., *Medical Women of America,* New York, Froben, 1933, pp. 58, 63.

applicants. Opposition to co-education seems to have been most intense in the conservative East, where the strongest schools were located. On the other hand, the Western Reserve College at Cleveland granted degrees to women as early as the 1850's, and the University of Michigan admitted them in 1869. The first real break in the East came with the opening of the Boston University Homeopathic College in 1874.

As soon as a few colleges became co-educational, some women urged the advantages of attending well-established institutions. Mary Putnam Jacobi, who was critical of the work given in women's colleges, insisted that admission to men's schools could be secured financially by grants.[16] This view was dramatically confirmed when Johns Hopkins accepted the funds secured by Miss Garrett in 1893, on condition that women be admitted on equal terms. The advantages of university connections were then being advocated as a means for reforming medical education, and certain women were impressed by this program. Thus, Emily Blackwell sought a merger of the Woman's Medical College of the New York Infirmary with Cornell University Medical College. When the latter refused this but itself admitted women in 1899, the former was closed as no longer necessary.[9] Similar action had meantime been taken in Boston and Chicago, so that by 1900 the only remaining woman's medical college was that in Philadelphia. After that year, one university after another accepted women, and by 1941, only 6 out of 77 medical schools were limited to men.

This being the case, many felt that there was no longer any *raison d'être* for a woman's college. But there was another side to the matter. In the earlier decades, those supporting women's colleges had had other reasons than vested interests for doubting the desirability of co-education. In the first place,

[16] Jacobi, M. P., *Papers of the First Congress of the Association for the Advancement of Women, New York, 1873*, pp. 168–178.

women were not always accepted on equal terms under the latter system. In some cases, they had to attend separate classes or sit behind screens. It is said that in the early days at Johns Hopkins, women students were allowed to examine men only above the neck—here male modesty entered the picture —with resulting embarrassment when the women were later assigned to men's wards. Even when these distinctions were abandoned, the advocates of separate colleges felt that they possessed distinct advantages. Notable were the greater opportunities which they afforded to women for internships, residencies, and faculty appointments. Although women have been admitted to the faculties of "co-ed" schools, particularly during the last two decades, this opportunity remains a limited one.

One other consideration which may have motivated the continued existence of the Woman's Medical College of Pennsylvania—apart from loyalty to alma mater—was concern about equal opportunities in medical education. Emily Blackwell and others may have assumed in 1900 that the schools, once they admitted women, would take care of all qualified applicants. In practice, however, the ratio of women in "co-ed" classes has averaged only from 5 to 10 percent; and one wonders whether the long-run effect of closing the women's colleges has not been to lessen the places which would otherwise have been open to women students. For those who believe that the country needs more physicians, such a trend would be of concern to national interests as well as to those of women. This was well illustrated during the recent war when, despite discrimination against women doctors in the Army, there was a sharp rise in demands for their services among the civilian population.[17]

So much for factors pro and con the admission of women

[17] *Women Physicians, Bull.,* 203, No. 7, Women's Bureau, Washington, 1945, pp. 5 ff.

into the medical profession. It has already been implied that opportunities for them were slowly expanding during the last half of the nineteenth century, particularly so after 1890. This was the result of the progress of feminism in general, and of advantages gained within medicine in particular. The first period in this story might be set between 1850 and 1870, when the women's schools in Philadelphia, New York, Chicago, and Boston were struggling for existence, and when the first women's hospitals were established. The early years were most difficult, when the schools were located in old buildings without equipment and the faculties consisted of such men as were willing to serve.

As soon as classes were graduated, certain of their members added to the staffs as professors and deans; and this made possible more enthusiastic teaching and competent administration. One may well pay tribute to both the courage and resourcefulness of these early leaders, such as Ann Preston in Philadelphia and Emily Blackwell in New York. Medical practice in itself was not an easy life; and these women added to it the tasks of teaching and administration at a time when their institutional resources were most inadequate. These were the days, according to legend, when a professor, after seeing patients in a small ward, might have to hurry to the kitchen to help prepare their food.

By 1870 it was clear that women in medicine had come to stay, but there remained much uncertainty as to their status. The next twenty years were ones of slow but continuous growth in the resources of the women's schools and in the numbers of their graduates. Teaching was improved by expanding the small faculties, by securing access to general clinics, and by enlarging women's hospitals. The Woman's Medical College of Pennsylvania kept pace with advancing science after 1890 by introducing laboratory work in physiology and bacteriology. Like most medical schools of the period, this College had practically no endowment and no aid from the state, medical science not yet having proved so useful as to elicit from a practical-minded society either private or public support.[18] Since all professors were engaged in private practice, however, the College did not have to worry about salaries; and laboratory facilities were as yet relatively inexpensive. Had the equipment of a medical school then been half as costly as it is today, these women's colleges probably could not have been established. As it was, they were able like other institutions to struggle on with the support of tuition fees. Occasional gifts were received for special purposes, such as the Jeanes fund which enabled the College here to move to its more substantial quarters on North College Avenue in 1875.

The women's schools realized the need for improving their position by performance rather than by argument. They were therefore anxious from the start to demonstrate the success of their graduates. In 1881 Dean Rachel Bodley of the Woman's Medical College reported that 276 had taken the degree in the course of 30 years, and that 189 had replied to her questionnaires. Most of the latter (109) were devoting themselves to obstetrics or gynecology or to a combination of these with general practice. Only three reported themselves as surgeons. The average income was almost $3,000 a year, which was not bad in view of the current value of the dollar. Over one-third were members of medical societies. On the whole this was an encouraging report for the oldest and largest of the women's medical colleges.[19]

Dean Bodley did not give the location of the graduates, but most of them were apparently practicing in northern cities. Few seem to have invaded conservative rural areas. A number

[18] Shryock, R. H., *American Medical Research: Past and Present,* New York, Commonwealth Fund, 1947, pp. 39 ff.
[19] Marshall, C., "The Woman's Medical College of Pennsylvania: a History," *Virginia M. Semi-Monthly,* Jan. 27, '99.

had embarked, however, on a more adventurous career in the Orient. Reflecting the religious idealism of early feminist circles, they combined good works with grace as medical missionaries in India and China. Through their influence, oriental students appeared at the College in Philadelphia in the 1880's, and have continued to do so ever since.[15] The College also welcomed a few Negro students, a group which was in a peculiarly difficult position because it had to face race in addition to sex prejudice.

In 1900 Dean Clara Marshall made a report similar to that of Dean Bodley in 1881. She observed that the students were now "younger and better" than in the old days. By this time a State Medical Board had been set up (1892) and Dr. Marshall proudly announced that all her graduates had passed its examinations in the preceding year. Incidentally, she added a new criterion of merit by noting the publication record of the faculty. During the College's first two decades, only one paper had appeared; but no less than 498 had been published during the 1890's. The Dean had hopes that the faculty would now engage in original investigations, a view which reflected the research enthusiasm which had been stimulated by the Hopkins school.[20]

It is of passing interest that both Dr. Bodley and Dr. Marshall found but few graduates who had abandoned practice because of marriage—only 8 out of 189 prior to the first report. The number of marriages was not given, but apparently most women found matrimony no bar to their work. At a time when there was general opposition to the employment of married women, the doctor had the advantage of her sisters in teaching or nursing because she was self-employed. The woman in private practice could not be

[20] Marshall, C., "Past, Present, and Future of the College," *Transactions of the Woman's Medical College of Pennsylvania Alumnae*, Philadelphia, 1900, p. 387.

dismissed.[21] Although medical women were proud of a few of their number who had secured salaried positions in schools or asylums, the great majority of their group was "on its own."

It is apparent that the 1890's were a promising era for the College, with the improvement of the student body, the introduction of laboratories, and the growth of the faculty to 66, about half of whom were women. In 1895 a small College hospital was founded, and in 1905 all connections with the Woman's Hospital were severed, presumably because of personal or administrative difficulties between the two institutions. This incident spread a rumor in the neighborhood of the College that women doctors were a quarrelsome lot; but this view need not be taken too seriously in view of the long record of analogous troubles within other schools. Separation from the Woman's Hospital made clear the need for an enlarged College Hospital, which was finally met by the removal to the present building of the College and its Hospital at East Falls in 1930.

Social trends were such, after 1900, that one might have expected enlarged opportunities for medical women. Population was growing rapidly, especially in the cities; and women were securing additional employment in many fields. The public demand for medical care was growing as a result of the increasing prestige of medical science. Feminism became more or less respectable and the medical woman no longer had to be so much of a crusader. Yet the increase in the number of women physicians leveled off after 1910, at the same time that opportunities for technicians and other auxiliary workers expanded. The number of women in medical work of all kinds advanced from about 7,400 in 1900 to over 20,000 in 1930; but within this total the percentage of physicians fell from 66

[21] Smith, M. P., "Restrictions affecting Rights of Married Women to Work," *Annals of American Academy of Political and Social Science*, 143; 255 ff., May, 1929.

in 1910 to only 40 in 1930. By 1940 the number of women physicians (including osteopaths) was 8,810, which was somewhat smaller than it had been at a high point in 1910. The percentage of women in the profession, moreover, declined from 6 in 1910 to 5.1 in 1940.

The same declines occurred among women in dentistry. Their number had risen from 25 in 1870 to 1,900 in 1920, but thereafter fell to 1,067 in 1940. The ratio of these women to the total number of dentists was 3.4 in 1920, and only 1.5 in 1940. In contrast, the number of women graduates in theology and law grew rapidly over the interval between 1910 and 1940, and their ratio to the total in these professions also increased. These trends can probably be viewed as delayed advances into the latter fields, however, for the rate of growth has been declining in recent decades. Moreover, the ratio of women in theology and law (about 2.5 percent in 1940) remains lower than that in medicine.[22]

The more or less stationary numbers and ratios of women in medicine over the last forty years may be ascribed to several factors. First, there was a drop in the numbers of osteopaths and perhaps also of homeopaths. Second, women may have had more difficulty than men in meeting the rising costs of medical education. Third (a factor already noted) most women's schools were closed after 1900, and co-educational colleges have admitted only small ratios of women students. Unless this procedure changes, it may be that the ratio of medical women to men has been stabilized at about 5 percent. There are still inequalities which must be faced; for example, the fact that marriage at 21 is likely to end a girl's potential medical career, while it has no such catastrophic effect upon a man. Half of the women physicians of 1940 were married, in contrast to only one-third of those in other professions; but

[22] Hooks, J. M., "Women's Occupations through Seven Decades," U.S. Dept. of Labor, Bull. 218, Women's Bureau, Washington, 1947, pp. 171–175.

the majority of the doctors probably took this step only *after* acquiring the M.D.

The apparent stabilization of the number and ratio of women physicians would seem to have implications for the one remaining women's school. This has at times enrolled as many as 10 percent of all medical students of this sex in the country. Presumably, if this college also had closed, there would have been an actual decline of women in the profession.

In concluding this discussion, I would raise two related questions concerning the entire story. First, why did the effort to admit women to medicine occur first in the United States rather than in Europe? Second, why did this movement, having originated here, encounter so much more opposition in the land of its birth than it did in most European countries?

Most social movements in the United States had a European origin; for example, the temperance and antislavery drives and even feminism itself in its general form. Why then did feminism in medicine appear first on this side of the Atlantic? One can only suggest clues. It is usually said that women received greater deference in American society, originally—perhaps—simply because they were less numerous in a pioneer population. Yet women were driven out of midwifery here and in England, but not out of this field in the rest of Europe. Perhaps their exclusion from any sort of practice here, particularly from that form for which they felt best adapted, was peculiarly irritating to ambitious women. There is no question, if European observers can be trusted, that unmarried women were far freer in the United States than in Continental Europe.[23] Once aroused, for whatever reason, American women were therefore in a better position to do something about it than were their French or German sisters.

But why, in view of these very circumstances, was opposi-

[23] Woody, T., *A History of Women's Education in the United States*, Lancaster, Pa., Science Press, 1929, II, pp. 386 ff.

tion to women so much more intense here? Again, foreign travelers provide a hint. They observed that, while single women were very free in America, married women were more completely dominated than they were in Europe.[24] Perhaps the men tolerated freedom for their daughters in the belief that they would soon settle down, but became alarmed at such a declaration of permanent independence as was implied in professional ambitions.

A more likely explanation of American opposition, however, is the very fact that the entrance of women into medicine here was associated with a strong feminist movement. This aroused resistance of like intensity, among many women as well as men. In Continental Europe, on the other hand, feminism in general was weaker and therefore inspired less alarm. Women seem to have slipped into French, Swiss, and Russian schools almost unnoticed. Except in the latter, moreover, the number of women students remained quite small and so was less likely to arouse opposition. One may conclude, therefore, with the paradoxical observation that the potency of the feminist crusade in this country explains both the pioneer character of the woman's medical movement here and the intense opposition which it encountered.

There are still Americans who believe that feminism was a well-meant but tragic mistake, that women have only been frustrated by their efforts to serve both within and outside the home. Current social ills, from divorce to juvenile delinquency, are blamed upon this double life which women have assumed or had thrust upon them.[25] It would not necessarily follow, even if all this were true, that the presence of women in the specialized field of medicine is undesirable. But many of

---

[24] Schönfeld, W., *Frauen in der Abendländischen Heilkunde,* Stuttgart, Ferdinand Enke Verlag, 1947, p. 138.

[25] Farnham, M. F., "Battles Won and Lost," *Annals of American Academy of Political and Social Science,* 251: 113 ff., May, 1947.

us will feel that, in any case, it is oversimplification to blame everything on the women. Feminism, after all, was a part of that larger trend which we term democracy. Both of these movements have involved difficulties yet unsolved, but both have also established values which we should be loath to lose. Not the least of these have been the achievements of women in general and of medical women in particular. May the Woman's Medical College of Pennsylvania, which is now the outstanding representative of this latter group, look forward to a second century of increasing usefulness!

MEDICAL THOUGHT AND RESEARCH

X

The Advent of Modern
Medicine in Philadelphia,
1800-1850 *

The historian can quote sources to suit his own purpose. It would be easy to portray the American medicine of 1800 as essentially forward-looking and progressive, if just the right evidence were selected to support this interpretation. This was indeed the view of contemporary physicians themselves, who faced the nineteenth century confident that American science had more than caught up with that across the Atlantic. In no locality was this optimism more apparent than in Philadelphia, then the capital, the largest city, and the chief medical training center of the land. None of the ordinary reproaches against the culture of this country, wrote Dr. Nathaniel Chapman of the University of Pennsylvania, can be applied to our science. In erudition, European physicians may surpass us, but "in penetration, and promptness of remedial resources . . . we are perhaps unrivaled. . . . It may be safely said," he added, "that in no country is medicine . . . better understood or more successfully practiced than in the United States." [1]

* Reprinted from *The Yale Journal of Biology and Medicine,* Vol. 13, No. 6, July, 1941—by permission.

[1] Editorial: *Philadelphia J. Med. & Phys. Sci.,* 1820, 1, 9. (Hereafter, this journal is referred to as Chapman's *Journal.*)

If such statements are discounted as due to patriotic feeling, one may still point with pride to other evidence of scientific progress in the Philadelphia of 1800. The city was notable for its institutional equipment, with the oldest hospital and medical school, a distinguished College of Physicians, and unsurpassed libraries and clinical facilities. Novel developments in chemistry were being pursued with enthusiasm; likewise, the relatively new experimentation in physiology and the latest developments in surgery. These subjects and institutions were in the hands of a brilliant galaxy of professional leaders, from elder statesmen like Rush and Barton to such promising youngsters as Physick and Chapman. Was it not amazing that Rush could anticipate so much that is now considered modern in medicine—as in his early "discovery" of the dangers of focal infection? Was not his concern with such fields as veterinary medicine and psychiatry—then generally neglected—well-nigh prophetic in nature? [2] To all such questions the answer would seem to be in the affirmative. If one stopped at this point, there could be no doubt that Philadelphia was already in the van of medical progress some one hundred and fifty years ago.

Unfortunately, one cannot stop here. There is another side to the picture, and this can be painted—again, if just the right materials are selected—in tones as somber or confusing as the preceding were bright and clear. As far as contemporary opinion is concerned, there was no end of both British and native comment pointing in this less happy direction. To begin with, much was said of the general cultural inferiority of the new nation. We have Sydney Smith's word for it that no one in the four quarters of the globe read an American

[2] For the development of medical institutions in Philadelphia prior to 1800, see the writings of Francis Packard, Burton A. Konkle, and Carl Bridenbaugh; on chemistry, the writings and collections of Edgar Fahs Smith.

book and—what is more to the point here—that the world as yet owed nothing to American physicians or surgeons.[3] If we discount such sentiments again, as due to lingering colonial-mindedness on this side of the water and to imperial attitudes on the other, there still remains the written record of the period. This may be presented in even more disconcerting forms.

One might just as well begin with Benjamin Rush, since his writings were more extensive and his influence more far-reaching than that of any of his colleagues in the Quaker City. Sooner or later the historian of the period is bound to stumble over him—I use the term deliberately, since the results are apt to be confusing. The same Rush who displayed the insights noted, also laid claim to many other achievements. He had, for example, solved all the problems of pathology and therapeutics in one final formula. As early as 1789, he had determined the treatment indicated for all the ills that flesh is heir to. Imagine the awe of his students, as they heard him announce the new medical gospel. Briefly stated, this amounted to saying that there is but one disease, and Benjamin Rush is its prophet! All illnesses, it appeared, were but "states" of one underlying condition; namely, of "excessive action" in the arterial walls. From this it followed that all sickness could be treated by depleting or relaxing procedures, primarily by bleeding and purging. The former was to be continued, when necessary, until the patient had been relieved of four-fifths of all the blood in his body.[4] Granting his premises, both the logic and verification of Rush's views seemed irrefutable. All could see for themselves that as his depleting proceeded, "excessive action" decreased; if the bleeding were continued long

[3] See James Eckman: "Anglo-American Hostility in American Medical Literature of the Nineteenth Century," *Bull. Hist. Med.*, 1941, 9, 31 ff.

[4] His doctrines are best found in his manuscript lecture notes, Univ. of Penna. Library. But note also his published medical essays; especially "In Defense of Bloodletting" in *Medical Inquiries*, 2nd ed., iv, 335 ff., 1805.

enough, the patient always did relax sooner or later. Rush was again forward-looking in this monistic type of pathology and therapeutics; but the future he here anticipated was that of the Christian Scientists, the osteopaths, and all the other sects that subsequently preached this gospel of one cause and one cure. True, he was in a sense the father of American psychiatry; but so, too, in his way, was he the grandfather of chiropractic.

It will be observed that the picture of medical progress prior to 1800 is becoming a little confused. It would aid in clarifying it if we could assume that Rush's doctrines were but incidental to his major work, or even that he himself was a unique personality in no way typical of the profession of his day. Unhappily, the most unique aspect of the man was his popular and courageous personality and the consequent extent of his influence. This guaranteed that his views, far from being peculiar, were spread over the greater part of the country by hundreds of admiring students. Some of these became in turn outstanding figures in such widely separated medical schools as those of New York, Charleston, Cincinnati, and Lexington; and these disciples tended—particularly in the West—to carry the master's doctrines to extremes. They could hardly outdo him in bleeding, given the anatomical limitations of the human animal, but they could and did improve upon his purging. Rush, in his day, observed John E. Cooke of Lexington, was "vilified" for giving as much as 10 grains of jalap, while now (1833) "thousands of physicians administer up to 100 grains." Cooke himself imposed upon his patients more than four tablespoons of calomel per day. He helped to build up a popular demand for such dosing, and there is solemn testimony that this reached a point at which rugged pioneers actually lived on bread and calomel in the place of their daily bread and butter! [5] Here was a phase of frontier

[5] L. P. Yandell: *A Memoir of the Life and Writings of John E. Cooke,* Louisville, 1875. Elisha Bartlett mentions the bread and calomel diet in his *Philosophy of Medical Science,* Philadelphia, 1844.

tradition which seems to have escaped the Western historians.

This is not to say that during all the years from 1800 to 1833, the theory and practice of Rush had gone unchallenged. It had been opposed from the very start, and nowhere more vigorously than in his native city. When he first advocated heroic bleeding and purging, during the yellow fever epidemic of 1793, it was new doctrine and more than one colleague denounced it. Prior to that time, local practitioners had been largely influenced by the Dutch master, Boerhaave, who allowed some leeway for the healing powers of Nature. But Rush had no confidence in Mother Nature, and insisted that she be driven from the sick room as one would a stray dog or cat. All depended on what the doctor did for—or to—the patient. Small wonder that the laity also took alarm at this juncture and expressed their feeling in print. One of them, the famous William Cobbett, attacked Rush as that "remorseless Master Bleeder." In the course of the controversy that ensued, the pamphleteer referred kindly to the doctor's system as "one of those great discoveries which are made from time to time for the depopulation of the earth." [6] Rush was even accused of deliberately misrepresenting the results of his treatments, and the Philadelphia Medical Society was still enthralled by discussions of this theme thirty years thereafter.[7]

Once the epidemic was over, the laity lost interest and medical men concerned themselves more and more with the pathological system on which Rush based these particular treatments. Could all disease really be reduced to one condition, and that one a state of "excessive action" in the arteries? The schism of 1793 continued. Influential pupils supported

[6] *Porcupine's Gazette,* Philadelphia, Sept. 26, 1797; and *A Report of an Action for Libel Brought by Benjamin Rush against William Cobbett,* Philadelphia, 1800 (statement of Edward Tilghmann).

[7] See T. D. Mitchell: "Vindication of Benjamin Rush." Ms. lecture before the Philadelphia Med. Soc., 1822 (Library of the College of Physicians).

the thesis in modified form for several decades. Even foreign observers spoke highly of his contributions, as when Adolph Henke praised his work in a handbook on pediatrics published at Frankfort in 1821, and Lettsom, of London, proclaimed him the American Sydenham.[8] On the other hand, physicians who had not fallen under his spell denounced the system as speculative and fantastic. Was this, in turn, the final answer? Did Philadelphia, at a time when it was peculiarly influential as the national medical center, just happen to be dominated by a theorist, by a reactionary who opposed the progress of real science? It would be easy to explain it all in this way, but unfortunately the plot thickens at this point. The very fact that Rush's influence survived so long in itself indicates that contemporary science was involved in the very difficulties which accounted for his extravagances. The controversy he precipitated was only one of many signs of what was then termed "the uncertainty of medicine."

It will be recalled that so little was known in 1800 about the causes or consequences of illness that physicians practically worked in the dark. They tried this or that remedy which authority recommended or which seemed helpful in personal experience, and claimed all things for their own cures. What one doctor asserted, another denied, and in consequence the public began to suspect that physick was not keeping pace with physics and the other natural sciences.[9] Medical men might, in principle, have employed all the methods of these

---

[8] *Am. J. Med. Sci.*, 1828, 2, 177. Formal defense of Rush's system began during his lifetime; see, e.g., John T. Reeves: *On the Medical Theories of Brown, Cullen, Darwin, and Rush*, Philadelphia, M.D. Thesis, 1805. The general controversy concerning Rush is presented in Nathan Goodman's biography, and in F. P. Henry (Ed.), *Standard History of the Medical Profession in Philadelphia*, Chicago, 1897, 199 ff. (This study was largely the work of Burton A. Konkle, according to statements inserted in the copy of the College of Physicians.)

[9] R. H. Shryock: *The Development of Modern Medicine*, Philadelphia, 1936 (Chapter on "Public Confidence Lost").

other disciplines, but as long as they focused on the cure of patients they could actually learn only by the slow process of trial and error. And even the "error" could be, and usually was, denied. No wonder that a pioneer pathologist in Philadelphia could exclaim in 1828: "The search for remedies led nowhere." [10]

What practitioners had to learn during the eighteenth century was that one could do little with most diseases until these had first been identified. The vaguest notions still obtained in this regard. In 1808, for example, Philadelphians were still dying of such interesting conditions as "decay," "debility," and of being "found dead." Ultimately, physicians would only distinguish between different diseases by viewing patients as data rather than as human beings, and many social and professional circumstances delayed this process. Efforts to classify diseases as one would botanical species, meanwhile, produced endless lists of symptomatic names which had little or no meaning. Hence, Rush's effort to reduce all these names to one.

Actually, of course, it was of small avail to substitute just one disease in the place of the eighteen hundred of the "nosologies"—to go from one extreme to the other. No one could deny the appearance of wide diversity in illness. Indeed, where the symptoms were particularly striking, a few "clinical pictures" had long been recognized. This was notably true of skin conditions like the great and the small pox. In such cases, the skin lesions apparently *were* the disease.

Now to identify a disease with local lesions was to adopt what was then known as a solidistic pathology. But this was quite a different view from the older speculative solidism, which assumed that all illness was due to mysterious tensions throughout blood vessels or nerves. Different, too, was the

[10] See John D. Godman: *Contributions to Physiology and Pathological Anatomy,* Philadelphia, 1825, 6 ff.

other traditional pathological theory, namely, that all diseases were "in the blood" or other humors. Both humoralists and solidists had at least one great advantage: if their theories were true, it was unnecessary to look further for explanations of disease.[11] But those who believed there were local lesions in illness must needs seek these out by long and difficult postmortem examinations.

This search was by no means an easy one. Autopsies presupposed hospitals, and these in turn presupposed large towns. When these were available, it was still necessary to overcome a popular aversion to dissections. Yet all these conditions had been attained to some degree in Dutch and Italian centers before the middle of the eighteenth century, and as a result pathological anatomy had been well formulated in Morgagni's classic work as early as 1761. The Italian leader realized that the essential problem in medicine was to correlate clinical observations with local postmortem findings in order to discover just what diseases medicine was dealing with.

This realization must have been imparted to some of the American physicians trained by that time in the best European schools. Indeed, there is clear evidence of this in a remarkable address given by Dr. Thomas Bond, upon the inauguration of clinical lectures at the Pennsylvania Hospital in 1766. As early as that year, Bond not only appreciated the general importance of the autopsy but envisaged clearly its essential value in checking speculative theories concerning the nature of disease. He recommended a procedure which was practically an equivalent of the modern pathological conference, and cited similar opinions from such earlier authorities as Boerhaave and Bonetus. The "clinical professor," he de-

[11] The speculative "systems" also had the advantage of explaining the diffusion of symptoms throughout the body, which they claimed the local pathology could not do. Localists met this by assumptions about a "sympathy" between the various parts. This was as speculative as the views of the humoralists, but served to justify continued research at the time.

clared, first comes to the aid of speculation. He observes and diagnoses. In case of death, he then "brings his knowledge to the test . . . by exposing all the Morbid parts to view and demonstrates by what means it [the disease] produced Death." He admits and points out his mistakes in diagnosis, as revealed by the pathological findings.[12]

Here was the very program which was destined, more than was any other one factor, to revolutionize medicine during the next century. It was thus clearly formulated in Philadelphia at the very outset of the most promising professional developments in the city. Why was there so little practice there of such precepts during the following decades, instead of the extravagant theories, the extreme practices, and the bitter controversies which actually ensued? The explanation lies partly in the nature of contemporary medical problems, partly in circumstances more or less peculiar to the American scene.

The most obvious explanation of scientific backwardness in America will be found in the idea of colonial isolation. "After all," it will be observed, "this was a new country." But such formulae oversimplify history, just as Rush's theories oversimplified medicine. Actually American culture was identical with, and therefore just as old as, that of Europe. Even in institutional equipment, Philadelphia at least was equal to most of the European cities in 1800. It was certainly one of the three chief medical centers in English-speaking lands, and was a world center of the Enlightenment. European physicians followed with some interest the writings of the Philadelphia "faculty" at the turn of the century, not only in reviews but in translations as well. There was, to be sure, some degree of isolation in the American setting; but intellectual contacts were fairly close and continuous after 1750, as the careers of

[12] Ms. lecture in the Philadelphia College of Physicians Library; reprinted in T. G. Morton and F. Woodbury: *The History of the Pennsylvania Hospital*, Philadelphia, 1879, 462 ff.

such local leaders as Rush, Franklin, and Rittenhouse attest. One must therefore search for more specific explanations of the failure to implement Dr. Bond's program.

Quite apparent was the survival of popular aversion to dissections in all Anglo-Saxon lands until about 1830, and in most American states long after that date. This must have handicapped autopsies, even in private practice, to some degree. There were no "doctors' riots" in Philadelphia as serious as those in New York or scandals as lurid as those of Edinburgh; but there is contemporary evidence as late as 1825 in the former city, that public feeling was a real obstacle in the way of systematic research.[13]

It is also to be recalled that American cities suffered to an unusual degree from certain disease conditions, notably from devastating fever epidemics between about 1790 and 1810. The yellow fever of 1793 in Philadelphia was probably the most terrible visitation ever experienced in this country. Such calamities may have inhibited systematic research, directly by distracting the attention of practitioners during the sickly autumnal period, indirectly, by concentrating their attention on the fevers in general. The latter influence was subtle, and was probably the more important one. To understand its implications, one must return to the problems which pathological research faced in all countries during the eighteenth century.

As has been stated above, a search for local seats of disease was not easy because it presupposed certain social and institutional facilities. But even granted all of these, the investigator encountered the most perplexing difficulties inherent in disease phenomena. Illness frequently carried no such tangible labels or identifying marks as in the case of skin conditions. Occasionally, a "clinical picture" without visible lesions was so

[13] John D. Godman: *Am. J. Med. Sci.,* 1828, 1, 491.

common and so striking as to be vaguely recognized as a sort of entity, or at least as a picture fairly distinct from all others. "Consumption" is a case in point. This particular condition, moreover, plainly pointed through its symptoms to unseen difficulties within the chest; and so Sylvius, by the middle of the seventeenth century, had been able to correlate cough and fever with tubercles.[14]

In many instances, however, it was more difficult to find distinctive symptoms or, having done this, to trace them to local lairs. Particularly confusing were such complexes as "dropsy" and the "fevers." The latter, indeed, were the real villains of the medical drama. Commonly endemic, or recurring in epidemic form, "the fevers" constantly forced themselves upon professional attention, and nowhere more so than in America. At autopsy, lesions were sometimes found, sometimes not; sometimes such as were discovered were in one part of the body, sometimes in another. There was too, the perennial confusion of cause and effect relationships. Was this inflammation of the intestinal membrane the basic condition —what would have been termed in the eighteenth century the "proximate cause" of the disease? And was the capillary distention observed in the flushed face at the bedside just a symptom thereof? Or was the basic condition really the capillary distention and the intestinal lesion but a symptom of *that?* It was tempting to accept the latter view, since all fevers apparently showed this circulatory phenomenon, and if this was the disease, the problem of all the fevers had been solved.

Now this was just the path which Rush followed when pressed by the terrible Philadelphia fevers for an immediate solution. But as he had simply put the cart before the horse, he was left stalled in conjectures about the general tension of

[14] Esmond R. Long: *History of Pathology,* Baltimore, 1928, 84.

blood vessels and the consequent unity of disease. The worst of it was that, like all systematizers, he had no need to go further. For if he was correct, why bother with the tedious and unpleasant business of autopsies? The problems were all solved.

It would seem likely that the influence exerted by such a "system" on Philadelphia medicine, between 1790 and 1820, had some bearing on the lag in pathological research which ensued there. Much the same thing may be said for other American centers. It is to be noted, in further confirmation of this, that similar results obtained in Edinburgh. Despite great professional prestige, Edinburgh medicine had come even earlier under the spell of tension theorists like Cullen and Brown—from whom Rush originally derived his ideas—and the Scottish capital also failed to become a primary center of pathological research. Perhaps this lag was one of the less happy influences exerted by Edinburgh upon America in general and upon Philadelphia in particular.

There was little that could have been done in the Quaker city at that time about the epidemics; although that little, in terms of sanitary reform, was attempted. But something might have been done sooner to divert the local profession from the influence of Edinburgh. We have not usually so viewed the matter, but it might have been better if American medical students in the later eighteenth century had continued to go to Leyden or had sought out Italy rather than Scotland. One would suppose that in Morgagni's Padua they might have been directed into the path that led to progress. The suggestion was actually made in Philadelphia somewhat later, when John Bell urged that Americans seek out Pisa and Bologna which, he held, were better equipped in all medical respects than either Edinburgh or Glasgow. Italians, he observed as a further inducement, were noted for the "engaging affability of their manners"—though just what this might imply as to

Scotsmen was not made clear.[15] The advice seems to have gone
largely unheeded. Only rarely did Philadelphians even tour
Italy. John Morgan, founder of the first American medical
school, did visit Morgagni, but the contact does not seem to
have determined the former's subsequent interests. It is only
rarely in fact that anything more than casual references to
Morgagni can be found in the Philadelphia literature during
the half century following his death.

It is true that Morgagni's works and other pathological
classics were available before 1790 in the excellent library of
the Pennsylvania Hospital.[16] But apparently their mere
presence was not enough to encourage busy practitioners to
undertake original work in this field. Nor could the addition
of Matthew Baillie and Bichat arouse them; they continued to
concentrate on the problems of daily practice and to debate
speculative solutions of the same. The first local medical
journals were generally devoted, after 1800, to individual
cases and cures. Thus, the volumes of the *Philadelphia
Medical Museum,* founded by John Redman Coxe in 1805,
were given over to accounts of yellow fever, surgical cases, and
notes on particular remedies. Rush, for example, announced
the discovery that consumption could be overcome by opium
and the use of an animal diet. Other contributions had such
titles as "Watkins' Case of a burn," "Otto, on nitric acid in a
chronic complaint," "Horse-shoe found in the middle of a
tree," and finally—a nice native touch—"On the Management of the Scalped-Head." It was, in brief, still the day of
cures and curiosities in American medical journalism.[17]

Occasionally a different note was sounded, though just how

[15] Some Account of the New Italian Medical Doctrine of Counter-
stimulants. Chapman's *Journal,* 1821, 3, 46.
[16] W. G. Malin: "Sketch of the History of the Medical Library of the
Pennsylvania Hospital," *Cat. Med. Library Penna. Hosp.,* Philadelphia,
1829, 8.
[17] These items are from vol. 3, 1807.

significant a one it is difficult to tell. Thus, in 1806, James Stuart published in this journal an account of the "Dissection of a Body that Died of Yellow Fever." [18] He declared therein that the value of a localization of disease had long been admitted, but that because of indolence or lack of time "two thousand years have left us without a study of the seats of many of the worst diseases." One's first enthusiasm over this statement is tempered by the fact that Stuart reported on only one case, and that he explained what he found in this as due to "a morbid excitement of the whole vascular system." This sounds much like Rush, and suggests that such occasional pathological studies as were made pointed nowhere because they had to be fitted into a speculative frame of reference.

Only some twenty years after the publication of the first great work in English by Baillie is there some evidence in Philadelphia of a serious concern with local pathology. Briefly stated, this evidence is found in both precept and practice. As far as practice is concerned, the first suggestion of systematic autopsies appears in 1820. In that year, yellow fever visited Philadelphia for the last time in a relatively minor epidemic, and postmortem studies were made on most of the victims.[19] Dr. Samuel Jackson, in reporting the results the next year, observed that they confirmed the occasional postmortem studies made during the epidemics of 1798 and 1805. It is suggestive that he declared it unnecessary to list the many individual cases in 1820.[20] More significant than these emergency examinations was the establishment, apparently shortly thereafter, of the "Philadelphia Anatomy Rooms," in which dissections were carried on in more or less routine fashion. In 1824 these were in charge of Dr. John D. Godman, who gave

[18] *Philadelphia Med. Museum,* 1806, 2, 300; 306.
[19] Chapman's *Journal,* 1821, 2, 23.
[20] *An Account of the Yellow or Malignant Fever . . . in Philadelphia in 1820,* Philadelphia, 1821, 77 ff.

considerable time to morbid anatomy and who therefore may be claimed as the pioneer pathologist of the city.[21] Godman's publications in this field (1824, 1825) appear somewhat primitive in comparison with the earlier European classics, but they do attest to original work and antedated Horner's text by several years.[22]

The influence of the pathological point of view on precept and practice after 1820 was quite marked. Most obvious was the general about-face in respect to all the attitudes that had characterized Philadelphia medicine in Rush's day only a decade before. Instead of complacency, there appeared a critical pessimism about the long delay in medical progress, and a conviction that the science was just beginning to make headway. We are at least two centuries behind the point we should have reached, declared Godman in 1824, if physicians had only kept to the path of pathological research inaugurated during the Renaissance. As it was, he declared, Bichat of Paris had finally started medicine on the right path in 1800, and it were better to preserve his work alone than all the other medical writings from Hippocrates to Rush.[23]

Samuel Jackson, strongly seconding Godman's views, analyzed the situation more carefully in his *Principles of Medicine* (1832). This was the first American work to give serious attention to "medical philosophy," and was to be followed more than a decade later with similar expositions by Elisha Bartlett and by Oliver Wendell Holmes. Speculative systems and nosologies, declared the Philadelphian, still operated on the level which the philosopher Compte termed "metaphysical." But pathological research, emulating the methods of the

[21] This was the view of his colleague, Samuel Jackson.

[22] *Anatomical Investigations*, etc., Philadelphia, 1824; and *Contributions to Physiology and Pathological Anatomy*, Philadelphia, 1825.

[23] *Contributions to Physiology and Pathological Anatomy*, 8; see also *Am. J. Med. Sci.*, 1828, 1, 376; 491.

physical sciences, would soon establish medicine on a "positive" basis.[24]

That Philadelphia leaders of the 'twenties agreed with these critical views, is well illustrated by their reaction against the speculative systems. It so happened that David Hosack of the New York school had revived, about 1820, a humoral doctrine in terms of "morbific lentors" and "acrimony" in the blood. This, observed various Philadelphians, is an "obsolete creed" now "generally exploded." They agreed that humoralism was not only unsound pathology, but that it led to absurd therapeutics as well. Medicines clearly did not enter the blood because they never could be recovered therefrom.[25]

The New Yorkers replied, implying that Hosack's revival of humoralism was in effect a reaction against Rush's solidistic conjectures. Dr. John Stearns, addressing the New York City Medical Society in 1823, declared that after all the humoral pathology had been standard for centuries. Then it was suddenly ridiculed and for the past fifty years a stigma attached to it. In the United States, he felt, this was all due to the popularity of one teacher and his university—presumably to Rush and the University of Pennsylvania.[26] But now the latter's "vascular system" had been itself suddenly extinguished, and in New York there was a justifiable return to Boerhaave and his humoralism.

We can now see that there was some reason in what the Philadelphians considered Hosack's madness. Not only was Rush's system conjectural in character, but no scheme of pathology could entirely ignore the blood and other fluids. Yet

[24] He quoted Dugald Stewart's *Philosophy of the Human Mind* in this connection in *Principles of Medicine Founded on the Structure and Functions of the Animal Organism,* Philadelphia, 1832, 10.

[25] See Chapman's *Journal,* 1821, 2, 297; 1822, 3, 302 ff.; 1822, 4, 344 ff.

[26] A Comparative View of the State of Medical Science among the Ancients and Moderns. Chapman's *Journal,* 1823, 7, 219 ff.

it will be recalled that a generation later, when the great Austrian pathologist Rokitansky attempted another revival of humoralism, he was immediately annihilated by Virchow. The spirit of the time was against the humoralists; for several decades the latent possibilities in blood pathology and therapeutics would have to stand aside while progress was made in local pathology. For although the humoralists were partly correct, there was as yet little evidence to support their views.

It is notable that although Hosack had reacted against Rush, the Philadelphian leaders themselves made little attempt after 1820 to defend the latter's system. There was a cautious admission that their former colleague had indeed carried things to one extreme, coupled with the implication that this was no excuse for going to the other. "Our school was right," observed Chapman, "in rejecting an archaic humoralism, and also in discarding the artificial nosographies. But we were wrong in our intemperate generalizations about the unity of illness. We had better hereafter identify diseases only in some approximate arrangement relating to the body parts, until we have become more enlightened in pathology." [27]

The new orientation in Philadelphia was plainly correlated with an increasing interest in French medicine. This can first be traced, rather indirectly, in the *Journal of Foreign Medical Science,* which had been founded in Philadelphia as the *Eclectic Repertory* in 1810. All the earlier volumes had been largely devoted to reprints from English and Scottish journals. Between 1815 and 1820 occasional articles by or about Parisian leaders began to appear. Rather suddenly, in 1821, French materials seem to burst into its pages. The volume for that year contained, for example, such items as "Laennec's

[27] Editorial review of David Hosack's *System of Practical Nosology,* in Chapman's *Journal,* 1821, 2, 404. I am assuming here that Chapman wrote these editorials where it is not otherwise noted.

New System of Diagnosis," "Exposition of the Doctrines of Broussais," and "Medical Letters from Paris"—the last a reprint from the French which suggests a little conscious Gallic propaganda.[28] Writing in his *Journal* during the same year, Chapman informed the profession that there had been a complete reorganization of the Paris hospitals during Napoleon's régime, and that this had made possible for the first time a really systematic type of pathological research.[29]

Samuel Jackson, a few years later, also pointed out that the French school owed its achievements to the "immense advantage" of its hospital facilities. Why, he exclaimed, have Americans not yet contributed to these studies? Simply because of "the paucity of our hospitals" and their "miserable mismanagement" from the scientific point of view.[30] Perhaps popular prejudices against dissection were still factors here. One suspects, however, that American hospitals could have been better managed if the local profession had demanded it. No doubt many practitioners, completely devoted to private practice and looking upon hospitals simply as charitable institutions, viewed the new French emphasis with suspicion. There was probably a vague fear that these "new fangled notions" would disturb the nice systems in which current practice revolved. As late as 1820, another contributor to Chapman's *Journal* opposed hospital studies in principle, as a "particularly dangerous form" of mere empiricism.[31]

Open opposition of this sort, however, seemed to disappear thereafter. In 1828, a reviewer in the same magazine could declare that there is no necessity "at the present day" to point

[28] *J. Foreign Med. Sci. & Lit.*, 1821, 1, 40; 365; 516. It is interesting to note that Godman had been editor of this journal before he began his pioneer research in the early twenties. He was thus probably one of the first in Philadelphia to follow the French literature closely.

[29] Chapman's *Journal*, 1821, 3, 383 ff.

[30] Jackson: *op. cit.*, xvii (note 20).

[31] Chapman's *Journal*, 1820, 1, 224.

out the "immense advantage" of institutional studies in pathology.[32] By that date, translations from the French were appearing in increasing numbers, first in England and shortly in this country, and the Library of the Pennsylvania Hospital also began to be swamped with works in the original. Meanwhile, Chapman's *Journal,* as well as the *Journal of Foreign Medical Science,* seemed to transfer almost all its attention to French publications. Of twenty-three foreign periodical items noted under "Pathology" in volume xɪv of the former (1827), twenty were derived directly or indirectly from French sources. Even English items were solemnly taken over from French reviews.

As was to have been expected, improvements in clinical observations at Paris aroused the same interest as did the postmortem investigations there. In a few cases, American physicians had described clear-cut pictures of disease early in the century. The account of hemophilia published by John C. Otto of Philadelphia (1803) was probably the first complete description ever given, and it seems unfortunate that its genetic implications were overlooked by biologists for nearly a century thereafter. Nathan Smith, of New Haven, provided an excellent clinical account of "typhus" (typhoid) in 1824, and had for years before this stressed the importance of exact clinical descriptions.[33] Smith seems to have been "ahead of his times" in this country, however, and it required foreign contacts to further the general adoption of his specific approach.

One must also remember that French methods called for more searching clinical examinations than had heretofore been customary. The local orientation encouraged methodo-

[32] *Am. J. Med. Sci.,* 1828, 1, 409. (The name of Chapman's *Journal* was changed to this title that year.)

[33] On Otto, see E. B. Krumbhaar's article in *Dict. Am. Biog.,* 1934, 14, 109; on Smith, *ibid.,* 1935, 17, 326.

logical improvements all along the line, as physicians strove to find exactly where symptoms were, or in what form or to what degree they had developed. One begins to hear of stethoscopes in Philadelphia during the 'twenties. Godman complained in 1824 that they were not being used extensively as yet. Just when thermometers and pulse-timing began to be regularly employed is not clear. There was undoubtedly a long delay, which seems curious in view of the simplicity of the procedures involved. Clinical thermometers were available at least by the 'forties, but we have W. W. Keen's word for it that few were in use at the time of the Civil War.[34]

Another phase of the improvement of clinical observation was Louis' introduction, about 1830, of the so-called "arithmetical method." Philadelphians had been given a broad hint in this direction as early as 1800, when William Cobbett had cited the local bills of mortality to prove that Rush was killing patients rather than curing them.[35] Unfortunately, practitioners had ignored the suggestion, either because of the source and the vagueness of the data, or because they themselves could not appreciate its possibilities. By 1830, increasing interest in the use of statistics in public hygiene—which had been under way for more than a century—had prepared the medical mind for Louis' use of actual clinical statistics. Thus Gouverneur Emerson, of Philadelphia, declared in 1828 that statistics were not only useful in describing public health conditions, but could also be employed to check the value of various systems of treatment.[36] Such views afforded a receptive background for the introduction of Louis' procedures during the 'thirties, after which time the use of simple clinical statistics was honored in principle if not in practice.[37]

[34] *Medical Research and Human Welfare*, Boston, 1917, 18.
[35] *Rush-Light*, New York, 1800, 49.
[36] "Medical Statistics . . . Showing the Mortality in Philadelphia, etc.," *Am. J. Med. Sci.*, 1828, 1, 116 ff.
[37] Samuel Jackson: *Address to the Medical Graduates of the University of Pennsylvania*, Philadelphia, 1840, 29.

Meanwhile, the interest in gross pathology stimulated by the French school brought about certain other changes in American attitudes. In the place of the patriotic complacency of 1800, there appeared in Philadelphia an implied recognition of the superiority of European medicine. Perhaps this was easier to swallow in the case of the French than of the British brand, because of the undercurrent of dislike for things British that continued to circulate in post-Revolutionary America. British editors encouraged this feeling, in turn, by occasional caustic criticisms of American medicine. This semi-political factor may have facilitated the *rapport* with Paris. Despite enthusiastic recognition of Bright's hospital reports and also those from Dublin after 1828, there continued to be considerable criticism of British medicine.[38]

This was encouraged, moreover, by another shift in attitudes implicit in what might be termed the pro-French movement. Instead of the pride in American practice which even Chapman exhibited, clinical and pathological checks encouraged critical uncertainty in therapeutics. Despite Rush's reaction, there had always been some interest in Philadelphia in the "self-limitation" of disease. Adam Kuhn had treated cases of delirium tremens by shutting them in closets and letting Nature do the rest. When the first inklings of French "nihilism" appeared, leading Americans first resisted the view but gradually came to accept it.[39] By 1840, Samuel Jackson could declare that "the least important part of the science . . . is the dosing of patients with medicine." He felt that "the highest art" often consisted of amusing the patients, and in giving them confidence through the use of imaginary remedies while Nature provided the real cure.[40] French skepticism thus found expression in Philadelphia just

[38] See, e.g., Chapman's *Journal*, 1820, 1, 423; Eckman: *op. cit.*, 35 ff.
[39] Edward H. Clark: *A Century of American Medicine*, Philadelphia, 1876, 45; 46.
[40] *Address to the Medical Graduates of the University of Pennsylvania*, Philadelphia, 1840, 11.

as it did in Vienna; but apparently it made way more slowly in Britain. At any rate, American critics scorned the practice of "those hard-dosing Islanders" on that ground. In all lands, of course, it took time for new light to penetrate the nooks and crannies of every-day practice.

The rapid absorption of Gallic ideas had one somewhat unfortunate consequence; namely, the temporary enthusiasm for the doctrines of Broussais.[41] While this leader did much to attract American attention to Paris during the 'twenties—he was a more spectacular person than Bichat—his influence was bound to be a confusing one. Broussais can be interpreted as a sort of transition link between the localized pathology and the older speculative systems. He led in the move to find local lesions in the fevers; but since these were frequently discovered in the gastrointestinal membranes, he jumped to the conclusion that all fevers were so located. In a word, he made an oversimplified "system" of local lesions themselves, and became as dogmatic about this particular short-cut as the older systematizers had ever been about their more generalized speculations. Actually, Broussais had been preceded down this path by an English authority, Clutterbuck, who in 1808 had announced that all fevers were due to lesions in the brain and nerves.[42] The French leader had also been anticipated by the New York physician Edward Miller, a former pupil of Rush, who declared, about 1812, that the seat of all fevers was in the stomach.[43] Chapman was much interested in Broussais, and pointed out rightly enough that the latter's emphasis upon "physiological medicine" was needed as a check on an exclusively anatomical approach. But as pathological checks on the gastrointestinal theory of Broussais accumulated in Paris, his influence rapidly waned in the states.

[41] See *Am. J. Med. Sci.*, 1828, 2, 174.

[42] Henry Clutterbuck: *An Inquiry into the Seat and Nature of Fever*, London, 1807, 22 ff.

[43] Samuel Miller: *The Medical Works of Edward Miller*, New York, 1814, 166.

The final stage in the approach to Paris was the migration of students to the medical Mecca. This is a familiar story in which Philadelphians and Bostonians played leading roles. It should be stressed, however, that it was only after the Americans had pretty well taken over French views in principle that they began the hegira. Associated with Samuel Jackson at the Philadelphia General Hospital during the 'twenties were two young associates, Gerhard and Pennock. The latter practically grew up in the new atmosphere and at Jackson's encouragement went abroad about 1830 to work under the Parisian masters. Prior to their return in the early 'thirties, William Horner had published in Philadelphia (1829) what is usually called the first attempt at a pathology text in America, and Jackson had brought out in 1832 his *Principles* already cited. At the same time another promising student at Jefferson, Samuel D. Gross, had absorbed the French point of view without benefit of European training, and departed to practice it in the Ohio Valley.[44] From his pen was to come the first real American text in pathology, which was published at Cincinnati in 1839 and which had no superior in English.[45] This work was destined to spread the gospel among the American profession at large.

Numbers of American students were already in Paris by 1826. Once there, they found that French practice itself was still divided between Brunonians and the followers of Broussais' recently announced "physiological medicine." Other foreign students were also appearing, notably the Germans who were forsaking the *Naturphilosophie* of the Fatherland.[46]

[44] Samuel D. Gross: *Autobiography*, Philadelphia, 1887, 40 ff.

[45] Esmond D. Long: *History of Pathology*, Baltimore, 1928, 166.

[46] Some of the returning Americans, notably Henry I. Bowditch, wrote about their Paris training, but the Germans gave more specific accounts of institutions and procedures. See, e.g., S. J. Otterburg: *Das medizinische Paris, ein Beitrag zur Geschichte der Medizin, und ein Wegweiser für deutsche Aerzte*, Carlsruhe, 1841. For the German background of this story, see Paul Diepgen: *Deutsche Medizin vor 100 Jahre: Ein Beitrag zur Geschichte der Romantik*, Leipzig, 1923.

Neither Americans nor Germans were longer interested in Brunonianism, which represented in Paris what Rush had stood for in Philadelphia. Rather were they seeking training under the new school of clinician-pathologists—Laennec, Andral, Louis—and from them they absorbed further the critical point of view of which they had already learned something before going abroad.[47]

By the time Gerhard, Pennock, and other Pennsylvanians returned from Paris, the professional situation seemed encouraging. "Quakerdelphia" had attained a population of some two hundred thousand, and medical institutions had expanded accordingly. Available in "Old Blockley" and the Pennsylvania Hospital were at least the minimum resources essential to clinical and pathological investigations. The Medical Library of the latter institution still contained the largest collections in the country. Meanwhile, the development of new medical schools, notably Jefferson and Pennsylvania Medical College, provided what in the long run must have been a healthy competition with the original University school. Ever since its founding in 1820, Chapman's *Journal* had opened its pages to the newer point of view, and continued to do so after 1828 under the title of the *American Journal of the Medical Sciences*. Its subsequent career as the outstanding American journal is well known, and under the brilliant editorship of Isaac Hayes it welcomed the best in native medicine.[48] Under these circumstances, the young men returning to Philadelphia thought it feasible to "carry on" in the procedures emphasized in Paris.

Gerhard, following Louis' work on the fevers, found himself involved in the same problem that had faced his teacher;

[47] On the Paris school of the period, see especially Marcel Fosseyeaux: *Paris Médicale en 1830*, Paris, 1930.

[48] Edward B. Krumbhaar: "Early Days of the American Journal of the Medical Sciences," *Med. Life*, 1929, 36, 240 ff.

that is, the difficulty of distinguishing between these most baffling clinical phenomena in pathological terms. The outcome was the publication of his classic paper of 1837 on the distinction between typhus and typhoid,—a differential study whose significance was ignored in Britain but promptly recognized in France. The appearance of this original work seemed to indicate an actual transplanting of Parisian medicine to America. The new approach had taken root; it would grow slowly thereafter of its own accord on this side of the Atlantic.

Whether or not the establishment of French medicine in the United States implied complete scientific maturity here, is another matter. American medicine continued to be dependent in some degree on European science throughout the rest of the century. Philadelphians, for example, showed little disposition to enlarge upon the interests acquired in Paris. Even pathological research moved slowly, as a lack of proper institutional facilities continued to hamper postmortem studies. Krumbhaar quotes Agnew as observing, as late as 1861, that "the subject of post mortems was embarrassed [at 'Blockley'] by more formalism than would be necessary to . . . induct an Archbishop into his holy calling." [49]

In marked contrast were the activities of the Germans, who returned from Paris after 1830 in a mood to improve upon their former masters. This can be seen in their use of the achromatic microscope, at a time when texts used in this country still referred to microscopy as "a lost art." Ehrenberg's studies of the infusoria were reported in Philadelphia in 1833; while Johannes Müller's work was recognized in 1838, and that of Henle in 1840. But not one person in the United States, exclaimed Jackson in the latter year, is now engaged in

[49] See Krumbhaar: "The History of Pathology in the Philadelphia General Hospital," *Med. Life,* 1933, April, 10.

similar studies.[50] He ascribed this inertia to the "commercial spirit" of the age, which led in both England and America to a worship of wealth and accorded small recognition to intellectual achievement. Hence, physicians must look to practice for both income and prestige, and had no time for research. There were, moreover, no such facilities for advanced clinical training in America as obtained on the Continent. Jackson beseeched his students to follow the Germans in original studies during at least their first lean years, ere the shades of money-making closed about them. It is interesting to note, in confirmation of his views, that Gross apparently made his start in pathological studies largely because he waited in vain for patients for eighteen months, and improved his time meanwhile by reading widely in French and German sources.[51]

Within another decade, American students would desert Paris for Berlin, Munich, and Vienna, in order to "catch up" with what the Germans were doing. And within Philadelphia, Joseph Leidy was to pursue microscopic studies in parasitology of real value to medicine, while J. K. Mitchell reasoned intelligently on the possible animalcular transmission of disease. But by and large, neither American nor British scientists were to play much of a role in the next great step which Continental investigators were to take; namely, the development of medical bacteriology. Why were physicians in this country relatively slow in turning to microscopes and other laboratory procedures? Samuel Jackson had an answer in 1840, and there was probably much truth in his view. But other factors, some of which have been noted above, must also have been involved. One can only pose the problem here: its

---

[50] *Am. J. Med. Sci.*, 1833, 12; Samuel Jackson: *Introductory Lecture on the Institutes of Medicine*, Philadelphia, 1838, 20; and *Address to the Medical Graduates of the University of Pennsylvania*, Philadelphia, 1840, 15.

[51] Samuel D. Gross: *Autobiography*, Philadelphia, 1887, 40 ff.

ramifications would take us into many aspects of contemporary American culture.

It should be added, as a postscript, that this analysis of early modern medicine in Philadelphia makes no pretense of telling the whole story. Necessarily omitted are special phases of scientific development; for example, such significant themes as surgery and obstetrics. Much could be said of Physick's influence on native surgery, and Hodge of Philadelphia has recently been recognized as the outstanding American in nineteenth-century obstetrics.[52] There has been only a passing reference to the early research in physiology at the University of Pennsylvania, to say nothing of pioneer interest in chemistry. The doctor's theses accepted at the University's medical school were frequently devoted, both before and after 1800, to physiological investigations. While most of these were of a relatively simple nature, they do suggest something of the very interests that were later to lead to brilliant results in the work of Beaumont.

From the laymen's point of view, no doubt, the most important themes in any medical history relate to therapeutics and surgery. After all, what were the end-results of these scientific developments? Did they merely satisfy the intellectual curiosity of those who participated or did they lead to something of benefit to the society which made them possible? The answer is not entirely encouraging, if one considers only the generation which witnessed the advent of modern medicine in this country. The best medicine of 1850 was, as already implied, becoming skeptical of the old remedies; "nihilistic" at a time when it was just beginning to find new drugs with which to replace them.

[52] See the papers by Herbert Thoms on the early Philadelphia obstetricians in the *Am. J. Obst. & Gynec.*, vols. 29, 33, and 37; and Lewis C. Sheffey: "The Early History of Obstetrics and Gynecology in Philadelphia," *Ann. Med. Hist.*, 1940, 3s. 2, 215 ff.

It was, to be sure, of some value to discard the more dangerous of the old procedures, and at the same time to reform the materia medica.[53] Philadelphia, with its pioneer College of Pharmacy (1821), played a leading role in this process. But there were psychical dangers involved, since the public felt that nothing was provided to replace its old-time remedies. Many turned to new systems like "Thomsonianism," which meanwhile had been expelled from regular medicine in a day when monistic pathologies and cures could no longer be tolerated. Henceforth, these "systems" would be known as "medical sects." Even quackery, about to be glorified by national advertising and distribution, benefited somewhat in the process.[54] Philadelphia had its share of quack nostrums and of quackish institutions.

Nevertheless, the very period after 1830 when the public became somewhat skeptical about medicine, was actually the most revolutionary and promising in the whole history of the medical sciences. Modern surgery was largely made possible by the local pathology that became dominant after 1830, for how could it have ever flourished under the dominance of humoralism? After all, one could hardly operate on the blood or the bile. In like manner, bacteriologists could never have begun their search for the causes of disease until the latter had been identified and to some extent differentiated. Bacteriology carried the whole approach of the pathology of 1840 to its logical conclusion, by adding to the discovery of specific lesions the revelation of specific causes and cures.

[53] Bleeding was occasionally practiced by older physicians for all sorts of conditions as late as about 1875, but had then become moderate and was much opposed by the younger men. For a contemporary argument, see R. H. Shryock (ed.): *Letters of Richard D. Arnold, 1808–1876: First Secretary of the American Medical Association* (Papers of Trinity Col. Hist. Soc., xviii–xix), Durham, N.C., 1929, 135 ff.
[54] R. H. Shryock: "Cults and Quackery in American Medical History," *Proc. Middle States Asso. of Hist. . . . Teachers,* 1939, 37, 24 ff.

The public, of course, was most impressed by these latter-day developments, and so has been inclined to view Pasteur and Koch, rather than Bichat and Virchow, as the founders of modern medicine. Americans all remember the discovery of anesthesia; but have long since forgotten Gerhard and Pennock, and think of Holmes only as an autocrat at the breakfast table. The flowering of a science is more attractive, more exciting than its root stage, and so medical popularizers have encouraged this same point of view. No one is likely to dramatize postmortem examinations, or to make a "movie" of Godman at the dissection table. It would seem to be the obligation, therefore, of the serious student to place these stages of medical advance in their true perspective.

This observation is not intended as a deprecation of the brilliant achievements of the later bacteriology and surgery. Nor does it imply uncritical approval of every aspect of the medical trends of 1815–1850. The whole specific approach of that era inevitably tended toward a neglect of non-specific elements in disease.[55] This neglect was hardly more than latent in the science of 1830, but would become more marked in the bacteriological age of 1890. By that time, physicians had largely forgotten older interests in such non-specific factors as psycho-somatic relationships, individual "constitutions," and even the surrounding social and cultural circumstances. But it is difficult to see how the whole advent of modern medicine under discussion could have taken any other course, at the time, than the use of the specific conceptions actually employed. Non-specific studies could—and did—accomplish much in dealing with certain diseases, but would never have opened the way to some of the most important fields in contemporary science.

[55] Dr. Iago Galdston recently read an interesting paper on this theme before the Philadelphia College of Physicians, published in the *Transactions* of the College, ser. 4, v. 9, 1941, 25–34.

This suggests a final note on the extent to which the specific approach of 1850 was actually paralleled by non-specific work in such a field as public hygiene. This made considerable headway before it was affected by either pathology or bacteriology. Typhus and malaria, for example, were brought under a considerable degree of control by the generalized concepts involved in "sanitary reform." The movement gained early headway in Philadelphia as a result of the yellow fever epidemics, and the city was unusual among the larger American towns in that its mortality rate fell somewhat during the second quarter of the nineteenth century.[56] It was urged in the city, before 1830, that a national sanitary convention should be called at which the various states could be represented.[57] Wilson Jewell, of the local Board of Health, finally provided leadership in this direction, and through his initial efforts the first American public health association was inaugurated in the years just preceding the Civil War.[58]

One must take leave of the Quaker city. Picture it, during that year of 1847, when a small gathering assembled there to form the American Medical Association. Since scientific progress seemed by this time fairly well assured, it was now the question of adequate professional standards that was most pressing. Not only did the city act as host for this body, but the latter repaid the compliment by giving all the offices of the new organization to men teaching in or trained by the University of Pennsylvania. Whether or not such an administrative monopoly was wise, it was at least a recognition of the dawn of modern medicine and of modern professional standards in the nation's former capital.

[56] F. L. Hoffman: "American Mortality Progress during the Last Half Century" in M. P. Ravenel (ed.): *A Half Century of Public Health,* New York, 1921, 103.

[57] See, "R. E. G." in *Am. J. Med. Sci.,* 1828, 1, 180 ff.

[58] R. H. Shryock: "The Early American Public Health Movement," *Am. J. Pub. Health,* 1937, 27, 965 ff.

XI

Benjamin Rush
from the Perspective
of the Twentieth Century *

It has recently been observed that "One often hears and sees Rush's name mentioned, but in a few tiresomely repeated connections; as a man and as a writer he is little known." [1] This is doubtless true so far as the general public is concerned: in contrast to his friends John Adams and Jefferson, Rush has been largely forgotten even by the well-informed. This may be explained, in some measure, by the political emphasis which characterized American historical writing until recent decades. Despite some interesting adventures in public office, Rush was never a major political figure; hence he was neglected by writers primarily interested in constitutions, parties, and affairs of state.

During the present century, scholars concerned with special phases of American history, notably with educational and literary developments, [2] began to give Rush serious attention; and as the interests of general historians broadened, they

* Reprinted from *Transactions & Studies of the College of Physicians of Philadelphia*, 4 Ser., Vol. 14, No. 3, December, 1946—by permission.

[1] Lyman H. Butterfield, *Year Book* of the Amer. Phil. Soc., 1945, p. 191.

[2] As in Ellis P. Oberholtzer, *The Literary History of Philadelphia* (Phila., 1906); and the careful study by Harry G. Good, *Benjamin Rush and His Services to American Education* (Berne, 1918).

noted his contributions to social reform.[3] In 1934 Nathan Goodman brought out the first full-length biography, which presented the whole man "vigorous in mind and body, and heroic in stature." [4] During the last few years, renewed interest has been manifested by literary historians. Notable is the current work of L. H. Butterfield, who, in cooperation with the American Philosophical Society, is preparing an edition of selected correspondence and also a Union Catalogue which will provide the first systematic guide to Rush's voluminous writings.[5] It seems likely, therefore, that Rush will receive wider attention in the future from scholars at large.

We are not primarily concerned here, however, with the rediscovery of the man by general and literary historians. In contrast with such writers, physicians and medical historians never forgot the Philadelphia leader, and comments on him have continued to appear ever since his death in 1813. An interesting essay could be prepared on the history of this literature *about* Rush; and this might throw light on changing medical perspectives over the years, as well as on the physician himself. One can only suggest the features that such an essay might assume. It would relate, first, to the often controversial contemporary writings; next to the eulogies of 1813; then to more basic criticisms appearing after 1820, which swelled to a chorus of condemnation during the '40's and '50's. Unfavorable mid-century reactions reflected the growing influence of French medicine in America, which repudiated nearly everything for which Rush had stood. These reactions were typical of most professional appraisals until our own time, save as these were tempered, in the case of Philadelphia critics, by a natural pride in a great local citizen.

A more balanced view became possible during the present century, as medicine returned in some degree to eighteenth-

[3] E.g., John Krout, *The Origins of Prohibition* (N.Y., 1925).
[4] Univ. of Penna. Press, Preface.
[5] Note 1, above, 190 ff.

century concepts. The attention recently accorded his work in psychiatry affords an obvious illustration of this renaissance of appreciation.[6] In certain respects, Rush's views no longer seem so strange to present medical thinkers as they did to those of 1850.

Yet even during recent decades one still encounters those extremes of opinion, those sharp contrasts of censure and praise, which characterized earlier writings. During the first half of the last century, there had been such divergent opinions as those of Dr. Elisha Bartlett and (somewhat earlier) of Dr. Lettsom of London. The former made the acid observation that there was more "utter nonsense and unqualified absurdity" in Rush's works than in the whole vast compass of medical literature;[7] while Lettsom went to the other extreme in claiming that the Philadelphian combined judgment and sagacity "in almost unprecedented degree."[8] Similarly extreme contrasts of opinion appeared as late as the 1920's and '30's. Dr. Victor Robinson, for example, observed in 1929 that "the career of Rush proves that . . . a physician with a facile pen may leave behind him several volumes entitled 'Medical Inquiries and Observations'—and not one page of scientific value. . . . There are few medical writers, and certainly none of celebrity, whose works are less worthy of perusal today than those of Rush."[9] Yet only a few years later Dr. Goodman claimed that Rush was extraordinarily successful in his treatments, and that he anticipated modern medicine in many ways.[10]

[6] See, e.g., Clifford B. Farr, "Benjamin Rush and American Psychiatry," *Amer. Jour. Psychiatry*, Centennial issue, 1944; R. H. Shryock, "The Psychiatry of Benjamin Rush," *ibid.*, vol. 101 (Jan. 1945).

[7] *The Philosophy of Medical Science* (Phila., 1844), 225.

[8] *Recollections of Dr. Rush* (Lon., 1815), 12 ff.

[9] *Medical Life*, vol. 36 (Sept., 1929), 445, 447.

[10] *Benjamin Rush*, 235, 254, etc. References to various opinions of Rush are appended to this work, and also to the author's article on Rush in the *Dict. of Amer. Biog.* Dr. Butterfield's finding lists will doubtless add more.

Such conflicting opinions, persisting over so long a period, suggest that we are dealing here not only with changing scientific perspectives but also with an unusually positive personality. This personality was so sincere and devoted, and yet so self-assured and aggressive withal, that it has continued to make friends and enemies throughout these many years. Hence there remains room for honest differences of opinion about Rush the man.

It should be possible, on the other hand, to approach agreement concerning the doctor's theory and practice—as measured by the science of his day—and to evaluate his place in American medical history. Subjective reactions to his personality have no place in such an analysis, which relates to what may be well viewed as the most important aspect of Rush's career. Certainly the "American Sydenham" was first and foremost a physician. Important as were his political, social, and literary contributions, he was primarily devoted to medicine. In this field alone was he *the* outstanding national leader. In practice, he seems to have viewed his political and social activities as those which any public-spirited physician should undertake; that is, these activities were incidental to the scientific career. Here there was an interesting contrast with his friend Franklin. For the latter, although declaring the primacy of scientific interests, seems actually to have subordinated them to public affairs.

For the sake of simplicity, the analysis of Rush's medical work may be limited to the well-rounded theory and practice of his later years—which means primarily the period following the great yellow fever epidemic of 1793. An analysis of his earlier views and of how and why these changed would not be without interest; but it was the final "system" which became the subject of controversy and on which Rush staked his permanent reputation.

Most basic to an understanding of this system was his

theory of pathology, or of what he termed the "proximate cause" of disease. He began by claiming that all fevers resulted from (1) a predisposing debility; (2) a stimulus which was the immediate, inciting cause, operating upon a debilitated body to produce (3) a convulsive excitement of "excessive action" in the walls of the blood vessels. This last condition, which related more to pathologic physiology than to pathologic anatomy, was viewed as the essence of the fevers. Subsequently, he declared this "convulsive action" to be the underlying feature of all apparently distinct forms of illness. "I have formerly said," he declared to his students in 1796, "that there was but one fever in the world. Be not startled, gentlemen; follow me and I will say there is but one disease in the world. The proximate cause is irregular convulsive or wrong action in the system affected. This . . . is a concise view of my theory of diseases. . . . I call upon you, gentlemen, at this early period either to approve or disapprove of it now."[11]

Stated as bluntly as this, the theory now sounds absurdly over-simple. Further analysis, however, shows that Rush was dealing here with basic problems which cannot be ignored in any concept of disease. Predisposing debility was analogous to the modern idea of "lowered resistance." It might be caused by fatigue, intemperance, faulty diet, emotional disturbances, and various other processes.

"Stimulus" (the immediate, inciting cause) was conceived broadly enough to include anything which would be listed today as an external etiologic factor. Rush did not distinguish clearly between circumstances producing debility and those acting as direct stimuli; thus he listed emotions—psychosomatic relations—under both headings. But note that he viewed

[11] Lectures on the Practice of Physic, I, No. 31; II, No. 1 (MSS., University of Pennsylvania Library).

the genesis of each illness as involving two circumstances—
the impact of an outside agent and the reaction of the body
itself. This view, later lost to sight in the preoccupation with
bacteria as the sole "cause" of certain diseases, is analogous to
the modern idea that the "cause" of an infection is really a
complex relationship between body cells and infectious
agents.[12]

Where Rush departed from views already held by some in
his own time, and more universally accepted thereafter, was in
his concept of the stimulus factor. He insisted that this was
entirely nonspecific in nature. All stimuli, no matter what
their character, were said to produce the same effect; that is,
the pathologic process of excessive action in the vascular
system. The body was capable of only this one primary form of
pathologic reaction, much as the optic nerve and visual center
react to any stimulus whatever in terms of sight. To be sure,
the pathologic process expressed itself in different symptoms
having different names—in a fever, a pleurisy, a dropsy, and
so on. But any one of these clinical pictures could be produced
by any sort of stimulus if the latter were strong enough. Rush
knew that certain etiologic factors (for example, smallpox
virus) seemed to be specific, but he expressly denied this. "My
view," he declared, "establishes the sameness of a pleurisy,
whether it be excited by heat succeeding cold, or by the
contagions of the smallpox and measles, or by the miasmata of
the yellow fever." [13]

This might be interpreted to mean simply that different
causative factors may produce similar symptoms—a truism in
itself—were it not that Rush denied specificity in pathology as
well as in etiology. All external factors were able to produce
the same symptoms because all of them led to the same
underlying pathologic process. This process, in turn, could

---

[12] Wiley D. Forbus, *Reaction to Injury* (Baltimore, 1943), 45 ff.
[13] Quoted by Goodman, *Benjamin Rush*, 232.

produce the variety of clinical pictures noted; though it is not clear in Rush's writings why it sometimes revealed itself in a dropsy and at other times in a fever. Whence came this basic doctrine of the underlying unity of disease?

Any attempt at explaining the origin of Rush's doctrine must take into consideration many phases of his thought as well as the chief medical problems of his day. There was no one, determining circumstance, but rather a convergence of influences—scientific, professional, and social—which led the physician toward this extreme position.

It is to be remembered, first, that monistic pathologic theories had been inherited from classical times. Stated very simply, these had ascribed disease processes either to the condition of the body fluids (humoralism) or to an alternating tension and laxness in the solid parts (solidism). The latter hypothesis was usually explained in terms of tension and laxity in the nervous or vascular systems, since these reached nearly all parts of the body, and any irregularities in them would therefore seem to explain the wide dispersal of symptoms—the fact that the ill man often seemed "sick all over." (It later proved difficult for the localized pathology of 1830 to explain this phenomenon.) In a general way, Rush may be identified with the persistence of this *strictum et laxum* tradition. Much interest had been displayed in it at Edinburgh where Rush was trained, and the immediate background of the latter's theory seems to have been an elaboration of this type of "system" by his fellow-student, John Brown.

Indeed, Rush was viewed in Europe as a sort of Brunonian, though he took pains to point out differences between this school and his own. Among other distinctions, Brown viewed "debility" as a lack of tone in body systems, and held that this was one of two main types of pathology, the other being excessive tone or action. But Rush insisted, as noted, that debility was not in itself disease but only a predisposition; and that the only truly pathologic condition was tension.[14] He thus reduced Brown's dualism of laxity and tension to the strictly monistic doctrine that tension alone was the substratum—the *ding an sich*—of all illness.

Why, however, after the brilliant advent of modern methods in medicine during the seventeenth century, was there this seeming reversion to classic speculations in pathology as late as 1800? This resulted, in part, from the very advances made in biological science during the interval between Harvey and Rush. So many new facts had been discovered that confusion was threatened, unless these could be interrelated by some all-embracing theory. At the very time that Rush was formulating his ideas, his teacher Cullen at Edinburgh declared: "For, when many new facts have been acquired, it becomes requisite that these should be incorporated into a system, whereby . . . the whole may be rendered more complete, consistent, and useful." [15] The Philadelphian took his master seriously.

No better illustration of the confused state of medical science could be had than the state of nosography—of disease identification and classification—in Rush's day. Through the centuries a number of striking clinical pictures had been recognized, such as "consumption" and certain skin diseases; but the first conscious, systematic attempt to identify distinct forms of illness came with the seventeenth century. Thereafter, the authority of Sydenham gave this search considerable impetus. Logically, it represented the first truly rational approach to medicine, for how could there be an intelligent study of causes and cures of diseases until the diseases themselves had first been found?

[14] Owsei Temkin, Comments on the German translation of Rush's account of Yellow Fever (MS., 1946, to appear in the *Festschrift* in honor of Dr. Victor Robinson).

[15] *First Lines of the Practice of Physick,* I (Edinburgh, 1796), 34.

Unfortunately, the only criterion which first appeared for disease identification was that of symptoms. This served well enough when these signs were obvious to all, as in the case of the "great pox" or of the "small pox." But the symptomatic classification of various fevers as "remittents," "intermittents," "continuing," "putrid," etc., was not so helpful. And as enthusiasm grew for identifying all possible symptom combinations as separate entities, long lists were prepared in nosography texts which amounted to only so many names. Rush rightly felt that these texts were most confusing, and desired some simpler scheme which would really aid the practitioner. He therefore swerved to the other extreme—from the listing of innumerable, supposed disease entities to the flat assertion that there was only one.[16]

There was, of course, a middle way between these extremes, one that eventually led out of nosographical confusion and thereby made modern medicine possible. This was the search for a localized, structural pathology. Once local lesions were charted and then correlated with ante-mortem symptoms, a basis for disease identification was secured which was far superior to symptom lists on the one hand or assumptions about disease unity on the other. Had the merely symptomatic nosography persisted, no one would ever have found either causes or cures for the long lists of names. Worse still, had the theories of Brown and Rush survived, there would never have been even a search for causes and cures, since there was nothing more to learn. Rush knew the one "proximate cause" of all disease and—as will be noted shortly—had the one means that would cure it. Accepting his premises, there was no need for further research. But the study of lesions by pathologists, and the correlation of these with clinical evi-

---

[16] See Temkin's quotation (*op. cit.*) on Rush's opinion of Cullen and Brown in this connection, taken from the former's *Sixteen Introductory Lectures* (Phila., 1811), 11 f.

dence, opened up the whole line of pathologic advance that led in turn to the development of medical bacteriology and immunology during the nineteenth century.

This more promising approach was getting under way in Rush's time. Morgagni had clearly indicated its possibilities about 1760, and shortly thereafter Dr. Thomas Bond actually explained them in a lecture at the Pennsylvania Hospital (1766).[17] Bichat and the French school were beginning intensive work in pathologic anatomy during Rush's later years. Yet the latter apparently was quite indifferent to all this promising research—rarely if ever does one find any reference to it in his writings. Originally interested in physiologic experimentation, in which his students did pioneer work in this country, Rush seems gradually to have become all-absorbed in practice. His later indifference to both physiologic and anatomic studies cannot for a moment be ascribed to laziness or inertia; he was a most intense worker, but one who by 1790 was giving nearly all his time to the bed-side and to the library.

I recall no specific statement by Rush which questions the laboratory approach, but one senses that he had little enthusiasm for it in his later years. He expressed the humanitarian zeal of the Enlightenment, and his one great purpose was to help his patients. This could not be done by turning aside to pathologic studies of no immediate value to therapy. He certainly would have repudiated the medical nihilism that ensued after 1830. Conversely, the discovery of a "system" that promised cures for all conditions must have thrilled a man who—in the tradition of the Revolution in which he had participated—hoped to benefit all mankind.

Although Rush seems to have inherited his major thesis from classical traditions, he was not necessarily aware of

[17] MS. lecture, College of Physicians of Phila. Library; printed in T. G. Morton and F. Woodbury, *The History of the Pennsylvania Hospital* (Phila., 1879), 462 ff.

indebtedness to earlier theorists. He observed that the first attempts to identify disease entities on a symptomatic basis had gone astray, and therefore cast about for some means to ending the confusion. Failing to see that the symptomatic criterion could be made really useful if correlated with pathologic anatomy, he adopted the ancient idea of disease unity,— perhaps without even considering at the moment that this *was* an ancient notion. He never supported it by appeals to authorities in a scholastic manner, but seems rather to have been impressed with the revolutionary character of his own ideas. Like other eighteenth-century theorists, indeed, he would have repudiated scholasticism; for the writings of empirical philosophers and the Baconian emphasis upon inductive reasoning had long since placed a premium on direct, independent investigations of Nature.

This fact, that the most speculative medical thinkers of the eighteenth century rendered at least lip service to inductive reasoning, raises an interesting question about Rush's own thought. Did he base his theory on something more than tradition—which doubtless influenced him even if he was unaware of it—and on something more than the pragmatic realization that it was useful in clarifying nosographic complexities? In a word, did he cite any actual evidence from which to induce his theory in the first place?

Here, it must be admitted, the writings are rather fragmentary and unsatisfactory. Rush usually just stated his premises and reasoned from them, using such dogmatic phrases as "my view establishes," and so on. Often he seemed to accept analogies as evidence, and was quite clever in employing ones that were apt and appealing in his day. Thus he suggests that the physician who thinks different clinical pictures are really different diseases, is as ignorant as a savage who supposed that water, dew, and frost are distinct substances. Or, again, he compares the theory of disease unity with noble monotheism in religion, while a belief in distinct diseases is equated with a superstitious belief in polytheism. Goodman declares that this was a very modern line of reasoning.[18]

Yet, imbedded in some of Rush's lectures, are hints of an empirical starting point. As might be expected, he took off on his speculative flights from a very circumscribed field of bedside observations. He had made the common observation that a flushed skin is associated with fevers. This was believed to indicate a distension of the capillaries. Since such "convulsive action" in the walls of these vessels was observed in *all* fevers, Rush concluded that it must be the essential pathology of these conditions.[19] Conversely, phenomena associated with some fevers but not with others—such as various symptoms or lesions—could not be essential to fevers as such. The underlying fallacy here was the initial assumption that "fever" was a sort of entity, but this was commonly held at that time. Once this was assumed, the reasoning was logical enough though just the reverse of that now employed. Rush would have held that the intestinal lesions, now viewed as the chief feature of typhoid fever, were mere after-effects of capillary or arterial distension; while we view as a secondary phenomenon the very capillary distension which he considered the essence of the disease. The doctor had the cart before the horse here; but in any case, he had them linked neatly together.

In attempting to explain the origin of Rush's "system," mention has now been made of the traditions behind it, of its pragmatic appeal in a time of confusion, and of the limited degree to which it was based upon actual clinical evidence. These explanations would be incomplete without additional reference to certain qualities of mind that lent themselves to the elaboration of ingenious hypotheses. The doctor had a

[18] *Benjamin Rush,* 235.
[19] Richard H. Shryock, *Development of Modern Medicine* (Phila., 1936), 28, 29.

keen interest in abstract and speculative questions, and was most at home in quasi-philosophical discussions. These qualities, combined with personal kindness, gave him an almost unique popularity with students; so that he probably contributed more than any other one man to making Philadelphia the chief national center of medical training.

Rush's imagination was stimulated by wide reading, and this suggested all sorts of plausible hypotheses—many of which were sound enough when applied to the social and historical problems of that epoch. Historians, who still fall back on their imagination at times, may appreciate these qualities more highly than do natural scientists. To put it more accurately, the historian is still likely to depend on his imagination in situations not admitting of final verification. He presents what seems the most convincing hypothesis; and unless quite careful, he soon writes as though the thesis were actually confirmed by the incomplete evidence available. Rush's thought operated on much this same level; that is, he began with some very limited evidence and on this basis formulated an hypothesis that was logical enough within its own structure. Then, since the thesis seemed plausible and promised cures, he accepted it enthusiastically and interpreted his clinical experience as verifying it.

All the steps in this chain of thought are sound enough until we come to the last—the failure to seek adequate verification. The treatment which Rush advocated was literally a cure-all—was good for what ailed you, since by definition the same thing ailed everyone. The procedures—which were largely bleeding and purging—will be discussed by Dr. Pepper. They followed logically from Rush's premises; for if disease consisted of vascular tension, then it could be cured by relieving that tension through bleeding. Anyone could see that, if the patient were bled copiously enough, he would relax—sooner or later! But such a superficial observation was far from providing a real verification of the soundness of the theory employed.

One should therefore pause to examine this weakest point in Rush's line of thought. How valid was his claim, for example, that he could almost always cure yellow fever by bleeding—provided the cases were not too far advanced—and that this proved the soundness of his underlying theory? In answer, it must be noted that (1) Rush's own clinical data were fragmentary—he kept no real statistics; (2) even if he had done so, the figures would have been based only on his own claims of cures. The idea of using "controls" to check a method of treatment does not seem to have occurred to him; and under these circumstances, his claims were suspect in terms of the *post hoc, ergo propter hoc* fallacy; (3) even if the physician *had* kept careful records, and checked his own treatments by the use of "controls," the limited experience of one observer was quite inadequate for the final demonstration of a sweeping hypothesis.

It is easy to show in this fashion that Rush's procedures did not measure up to present canons of scientific method, or to those which Bichat would have demanded in that day. Yet even here, one can feel some sympathy for the former's difficulties. The Philadelphian was by no means visionary in seeking clues in pathologic physiology rather than in pathologic anatomy; yet it happened that the first field offered more difficulty than the second in the way of verification. Bichat could verify his thesis that lesions were common to certain types of tissues with relative ease; whereas—given the state of physiology at the time—there was just no way for Rush to test whether a tension in capillaries caused what he viewed as mere after-effect in the form of organic lesions.

Hence he was under great temptation to seek confirmation by the only apparent means—the appeal to clinical experience. It is only fair to recall that innumerable physicians had reported, through the centuries, that bleeding did give excellent results in all manner of conditions. Doubtless Rush felt that the evidence in favor of his treatments—and therefore of his theory—was cumulative even if incomplete.

It is also to be recalled that he was no more careless in handling clinical data than were the great majority of medical men in his day. Perhaps a few individual physicians had suggested the keeping of accurate records, and had been prevented from doing this both by lack of time and lack of enough data to make it worth while. Large hospital services, bringing hundreds of similar cases under the view of a single clinician, were still pretty much in the future. Statistics and the calculus of probabilities were young sciences in Rush's day, moreover, and it was not until three years before his death that the mathematician Laplace called attention to the value of these disciplines for medical studies.[20]

Strangely enough, the first attempt to apply statistics in therapy which I have encountered is that of William Cobbett —an attempt made in the course of the pamphleteer's famous controversy with Rush. Cobbett had no real clinical statistics; but he went to the local bills of mortality to prove mathematically that the doctor was killing yellow fever patients rather than curing them.[21] In relation to the history of scientific method, this episode deserves more attention than it has received. While Rush was then in no mood to accept any suggestion coming from Cobbett, it is also true that physicians in general ignored this early appeal to quantitative procedures.

Within a decade after Rush's death, the French school had firmly established approaches to medicine which were the antithesis of his own. Research was concentrated on the correlation of structural lesions with associated clinical data, in

[20] *Théorie Analytique des Probabilités*, 3 ed. (Paris, 1920), 420 ff.
[21] *The Rush Light* (N.Y., Feb. 28, 1800), 49.

the effort to identify specific disease entities. This brought with it a demand for all the more accurate methods of observation—instruments, statistics—which Rush and most of his contemporaries had ignored. As a logical corollary, the whole theory of the unity of disease was repudiated.

This theory, to be sure, has been revived from time to time down to our own day. The thrill of finding the *one* pathologic condition, with its promise of one cure, continued to appeal to certain theorists and to many laymen. No doubt Hahnemann and the early homeopaths; "Doctor" Still and the osteopaths, and Mrs. Eddy and the Christian Scientists, all felt the same exaltation in proclaiming one cause and one cure as Rush once had in announcing his revolutionary "system." But the latter worked in a day when the weaknesses of this approach were not yet clear; whereas the others proclaimed their views when medical science had advanced to a position making them plainly untenable. Hence Rush was a great physician in good standing, while the others were excluded from regular medicine and became the founders of modern sects.

In summing up, the most serious criticism of Rush seems to be that he persisted in a traditional approach to the problem of disease, in a day when more promising procedures were already being adopted in European centers. While his reasoning was ingenious and generally consistent, his temperament and other factors were such that he pushed his approach to extremes in practice. Yet this does not mean that the praises heaped upon him were unmerited. He was, in some respects, a keen clinical observer, and note how his imagination served him in such a matter as the recognition of focal infection. His work in psychiatry has been duly appreciated in recent years, as interest in a psychological orientation in that field has revived. Here he was at his best, for the subject called only for clinical observation, and involved reasoning about matters that were abstract and obscure. His theories about local miasmas, as disease-producing stimuli in epidemics, were no more one-sided than were those of his opponents; and they had the added merit of encouraging the great sanitary reform movements which were inaugurated during his own life-time. His very indifference to laboratory research may be interpreted as the defect of his virtues; since it seems to have resulted from his earnest desire to aid suffering humanity, rather than to bury himself in investigations remote from the needs of his friends and patients. And though the influence of his "system" probably delayed such research in this country, he was only one of many clinicians who then and subsequently displayed little interest in laboratory investigations.

It has already been implied that, although Rush looked backward in his theory of disease, he was modern in the sense that certain of his eighteenth-century views have been revived during our own time. His concentration on "excessive action" in the vascular system seems analogous to the concern now accorded the whole "hyptertension" complex. (Incidentally, current theories regarding this major problem still divide along much the same lines that separated the two theoretical schools of the earlier centuries; that is, between humoral and tension hypotheses.) [22] Even Rush's doctrine of disease unity had the merit of viewing the patient as a whole—a merit that was lost during much of the nineteenth century when emphasis upon specificity was carried to extremes. His concern with psychosomatic relations is an excellent illustration in this connection.

Rush illustrates, finally, two other eighteenth-century traits or practices which were largely lost thereafter, only to be revived in recent years. These relate not to physicians in particular but to scientists in general, among whom Rush—with his wide interests ranging from chemistry to psychology—would certainly have arrayed himself. The first trait was

[22] See, e.g., Eugene M. Landis, "Pathogenesis of Hypertension in Man," Univ. of Penna. Bicent. Conf. on *Hypertension* (Phila., 1941), 9 ff.

this very versatility which was so typical of many seventeenth-
and eighteenth-century thinkers. At this point we usually
think at once, in this city, of Franklin; but versatility was also
characteristic of Rush, of Jefferson, of Benjamin Thompson,
and of William Charles Wells—to name only some of
Franklin's own countrymen. True, it was easier to be versatile
when science and learning were relatively non-technical.
With the growth of knowledge during the 1800's, progress
seemed possible only through specialization. But the resulting
divisions between fields must now in some way be overcome,
so that something of that earlier access from one area to
another may be revived. Rush's type of mind would be most
helpful today in what is termed "cross-fertilization" or "the
breaking down of departmental barriers."

The second practice which Rush well illustrated in his day,
and for which there is now a renewed demand, was the active
participation by scientists in public affairs. He considered it
his duty, as a physician and an intellectual, to take part in the
Revolution, and it was no accident that he became a signer of
the Declaration of Independence. Although he held no major
political positions, he gave himself thereafter to all sorts of
social reforms. In like manner the two greatest American
physicists of that era, Benjamin Franklin and Benjamin
Thompson, each became an outstanding public figure; the
one in his own country and the other—as an exiled Loyalist—
in Bavaria.

Subsequently, something of a divorce between science and
public affairs ensued. By the later nineteenth century, few
scientists were active in public life, and governments took
small interest in science—at least in English-speaking lands. I
need not labor the point of how all this has changed of late,
and of how scientists are once more becoming public figures
and governments are taking them seriously—or at least more
seriously than they did but a generation ago. The atomic

bomb only dramatized trends which had already set in in this direction.

The moral of all this is that Rush was more modern in many ways, as a medical man and as a scientist, than we might at first suppose upon dipping into his lectures and essays. The most famous American physician of his time, he did much to establish a great medical tradition in Philadelphia. Despite scientific and human limitations, he remains a striking figure in whom Americans in general and Philadelphians in particular may well take an unaffected pride.

XII

Early American Immunology:

As Formulated by the Reverend Cotton
Mather of Boston, 1725*

Little has been written about medicine as it existed in the
English-American Colonies prior to about 1750. Yet European medicine was practiced in these Colonies for well over a
century before that time. The reasons for this neglect of early
Colonial medicine are obvious enough. American physicians
of that period received no formal training, the profession was
unorganized, and there were no such medical institutions as
schools, libraries, or hospitals. The population was small; in
1720, for example, only four towns could boast of as many as
5,000 inhabitants. The few men who were at all learned in
medicine were not the apprentice-trained physicians but were
rather the generally well-educated government officials or
clergymen. Even these men wrote little in the medical field,
and that little was unpublished and of a fragmentary nature.

The chief exception to this rule is to be observed in the
work of the Reverend Cotton Mather, a clergyman of the
Calvinistic, State Church in Boston, Massachusetts. Mather
was a prominent figure there during the years between about
1690 and 1725. He is usually remembered now for his

* Estratto da "Atti" del XIV Congresso Internazionale di Storia della
Medicina, Vol. II (Roma–Salerno 13–20 Settembre, 1954)—by permission.

theological and historical writings, but was also much concerned with medicine and at one time thought seriously of practicing as a physician. He was, moreover, interested in many aspects of contemporary science and became one of the few Colonial members of the Royal Society of London.

Mather's medical thought combined theological, occult, and scientific ideas in a way which seems bizarre today but which was not uncommon in the seventeenth century. He ascribed all disease, for example, to an ultimate source in original sin. Although much of his writing now appears archaic, he kept abreast of the latest scientific developments of his time. He may therefore be viewed as a transitional figure who simultaneously looked back to the Renaissance and Reformation and forward to the *Aufkläkung* or Enlightenment. We are concerned here only with the forward-looking aspects of his medical thought.

Mather published a number of pamphlets on measles and on smallpox, sent reports on case histories and promising drugs to the Royal Society, and sought at times to advise the local physicians. But his chief work in this field was the completion, about 1725, of a general treatise on medicine entitled "The Angel of Bethesda." This *opus,* although never published and subsequently ridiculed or forgotten, offers us the only such treatise prepared in the English Colonies prior to the American Revolution. It was in part a scientific work, in part a popular manual for family use (domestic medicine). Although crammed with moralizings and lists of meaningless drugs, it is of great interest in two respects. It is unique in American annals in providing an integration of theology and medicine, and it is also the only American study of the eighteenth century which presents the animalcular or "germ" theory of the origin of infections.

Mather derived this theory from the writings of Kircher, Lieuwenhoek, and Benjamin Marten of London. He made no attempt to verify it by direct observations, but accepted it as best explaining many epidemiologic phenomena. In this respect, he shared the views of various Europeans who were then interested in the animalcular hypothesis. Mather was unusual, however, in that he applied the hypothesis to a new field—to what would now be termed immunology. This application came about in the following manner.

Medicine appealed to Mather, not only as a science but also as a means for helping his fellow men. He was anxious, as a clergyman, to employ medicine for the welfare of his parishioners and of his entire community. He particularly desired to protect the public from the diseases which were then most feared, that is, from epidemics of measles, diphtheria, and smallpox. Hence he was much interested when, about 1715, a Negro slave told him about an African practice of inoculating men with smallpox "virus" as an immunizing procedure. This interest was heightened when, several years later, reports of a similar folk practice in the Near East appeared in the *Transactions of the Royal Society*. The clergyman then decided to urge the use of inoculations whenever smallpox again broke out in his city.

Smallpox epidemics occurred, almost simultaneously, in both London and Boston in 1721. In the former city, at the urging of Lady Montagu, some twenty persons were inoculated in the hope that they would suffer mild cases and be protected thereafter against infection. This well-known episode is usually said to mark the beginnings of inoculation in the Western world. What actually happened, however, was that one or two deaths occurred following these inoculations; hence there was much opposition and no extensive experimentation with the practice occurred in England that year.

In Boston, meantime, Mather appealed to the local physicians to employ the same procedure. All but one of these men refused, condemning inoculations as both dangerous and irreligious. But Mather persuaded one practitioner, Zabdiel Boylston, to undertake this work; and during the next five months Boylston inoculated nearly two hundred and fifty persons. This was apparently the first experiment with active immunization ever carried out on a significant scale in the Western world. Mather and Boylston reported to the Royal Society that the inoculated cases of smallpox were usually mild and that the mortality rate among them was—at the worst—not more than two percent. In contrast, the rate among cases acquired "in the natural way" was over fifteen percent.

These reports were contested in London as in Boston, but they became a part of the evidence which supported continued inoculations in England, and from that country the practice spread gradually to the Continent. By the later eighteenth century, it became widespread and was made much safer when Jenner modified it by using cowpox rather than smallpox virus (1798). Thus, the experiments instigated by Mather and carried out by Boylston were the beginning of a positive type of preventive medicine.

It is usually assumed that early inoculations were merely empirical procedures but this was not the whole story in Mather's case. Like several contemporary Europeans, he formulated theories in order to explain why the inoculated "virus" usually produced only a mild case and also conferred immunity thereafter.

The clergyman's explanation of the mild reactions was as follows. In "natural" infection, he held, the smallpox virus first gained access to the body through respiration. From the lungs, the "virus" was then carried directly by the blood to the surrounding organs, where it did immediate, major damage. Serious illness ensued. But when the virus was introduced by inoculation, it was injected into a limb distant from these organs. It then had to make its way to the central parts of the body, and in the process was resisted by the blood or solid structures. Hence, by the time the "virus" reached the heart, lungs, and so on, it was weakened, or, as we would now say, attenuated. Only a mild illness then followed.

Mather thus assumed that mild reactions following inoculation could be explained entirely by what happened *after* the virus entered the body. His theory was vague but plausible, and it can be reconciled, at least in a general way, with modern views of the varying susceptibility of different body parts and also with present concepts of the role of the blood in resisting infections. Few contemporaries even envisaged the problem with which he was concerned. There were, however, several European physicians who also pondered the matter and they suggested another theory; namely, that the virus was weakened in some way *before* it was injected in inoculations. This also could, in theory, account for the mild reactions.

Mather went further than most of these early immunologists, meantime, in employing the animalcular hypothesis at this point. The virus used in the inoculations, he held, was probably composed of pathogenic microorganisms. He declared indeed, that it was this theory which led him to ponder the problems of infection in the first place. As he put it, this "germ" theory drew him "into new Sentiments about the way of its (smallpox's) Conveyance, and the Cause why tis conveyed but once."

The animalcular theory then led Mather into further speculations on the second problem which he here mentions; that is, on how inoculations produced subsequent immunity. His exact words were:

> The Enemy (the living "virus") 'tis true, gets in so far (into the body) as to make some Spoil; even so much as to satisfy him, and leave no prey in the Body of the Patient, for him ever afterwards to seize upon . . . the vital Powers are (therefore) sure of never being troubled with him anymore.

The use here of such words as "enemy" and "prey" was probably suggested by the assumption that the "virus" was indeed composed of living invaders. The meaning of the statement may have been that the "virus," once present in any part of the body, consumed all that was useful to it. Then, if a similar "virus" invaded the body at a later time, it found no appropriate substance remaining and could not survive. Hence one attack of the disease conferred lasting immunity.

Such speculation now seems a bit fanciful. More pertinent to modern concepts was Mather's realization that the animalcular theory held out great possibilities for chemotherapy. Drugs which could kill the pathogenic animalculae would be far more effective, he declared, than any remedies then in use. The animalculae must be entirely eliminated: otherwise, the few remaining ones would multiply and so continue the disease process. But Mather noted that such chemotherapeutic agents as were then available (notably mercury) were highly dangerous to patients as well as to microorganisms. The implication was that new and safer drugs must be found. Since Mather believed that different species of organisms would produce different diseases, one may also see here an inplication that the drugs needed would have to be of a more or less specific nature. But Mather made no specific statement to that effect.

It is surprising that a provincial clergyman should have envisaged both the promise and the difficulties of chemotherapy as early as 1725. But there is no evidence that his suggestions on this subject exerted any influence on contemporary medicine. Mather's enduring contribution was therefore not made in the field of therapy, but rather in that of preventive medicine.

In playing a part in introducing active immunizations into American and European practice, Mather helped to inaugurate a significant trend in later medicine. Inoculations against smallpox not only led into Jenner's work on vaccination, (which was simply inoculation with a safer virus) but also prompted inoculating experiments with such other diseases as syphilis, measles, and tuberculosis during the century between 1775 and 1875. After the latter date, as is well known, Pasteur and others finally established active immunizations on the same rational, bacteriologic basis as Mather had earlier postulated. It would seem, therefore, that the Boston clergyman deserves a place in the history of Western medicine as a whole.

XIII

The Strange Case of Wells' Theory
of Natural Selection (1813):

Some Comments on the Dissemination
of Scientific Ideas*

The indifference with which William Charles Wells' suggestion of the "Darwinian hypothesis" was received when first proposed in 1813, and the subsequent lack of recognition, are interesting phenomena in the history of ideas. Although this statement of the theory of natural selection in the origin of species was declared by Darwin himself to have been "the first recognition which has been indicated," subsequent historians have usually ignored it. This was true, until very recently, even of those specializing in the history of biology.[1] It is safe to say that at the present time, Wells' writing on this theme is still little known to scientists and almost unknown to general historians.[2]

* Reprinted from *Studies and Essays in the History of Science and Learning in Honor of George Sarton,* 1946—by permission.

[1] Note, e.g., E. Radl, *The History of Biological Theories,* translated and adapted by E. J. Hatfield (London, 1930); Erick Nordenskiöld, *The History of Biology,* translated by L. B. Eyre (1935). H. F. Osborn, *From the Greeks to Darwin* (New York, 1905), pp. 221, 222, however, recognized Wells' work as "the most complete of all the anticipations of Darwin." It may be that English-speaking historians are most likely to recall him.

[2] One of the few references to Wells by a general historian is that in Thomas C. Johnson, Jr., *Scientific Interests in the Old South* (New York, 1936), 3 n., p. 126. Two interesting papers relating to Wells' theory have been published in recent years; i.e., Conway Zirkle, "Natural Selection

One might have expected that pure curiosity would have made for greater interest in Wells. Other motives might also have led to the same end. National enthusiasm, which has at times influenced even scientists, would be calculated to revive this story, since here was a physician of American origin for whom great things could be claimed.[3] It is true that Wells has been recalled from time to time, but usually for his valuable contributions in physics and medicine rather than for those to biological theory.[4] Indeed this Anglo-American received high praise from distinguished leaders for his labors in these first two fields—both during his lifetime and in succeeding generations.[5]

Only rarely, however, has there been analogous recognition of the man as a biologist; and when this has occurred, it has quite naturally been coupled with indignation that he has been so neglected. Thus N. B. Jenkins, writing in 1909,

---

before the Origin of Species," *Proceedings* of the American Philosophical Society, LXXXIV (Philadelphia, April, 1941), 71–123; and Charles A. Kofoid, "An American Pioneer in Science, Dr. William Charles Wells, 1757–1817," *The Scientific Monthly*, LVII (Washington, July, 1943), 77–80.

[3] Wells was born and reared in Charleston, South Carolina; and although part of his school years were spent in Britain, he received his professional training in that city. Subsequently, as a loyalist during the Revolution, he moved to London and made his professional career there. See William Charles Wells, *Dictionary of American Biography*, XIX (New York, 1936), 644, 645. Kofoid, *op. cit.*, p. 77, first declares that the only American claim on Wells is his birth at Charleston, but then cites Wells himself as to the "lasting influence" of his professional training in the same city.

[4] See, e.g., Harry Keil, "Dr. William Charles Wells and His Contribution to the Study of Rheumatic Fever," *Bulletin of the Institute of the History of Medicine*, IV (Baltimore, 1936), 789 ff. A considerable bibliography of later references to Wells' medical works could be compiled from British and American medical journals, most of which is noted in Keil's article.

[5] See quotations in *ibid.*, p. 791. Dr. Ashley Montagu has called my attention to Tyndall's reference (in his "Belfast Address," 1874) to Wells as "long ago a favorite with me"; John Tyndall, *Fragments of Science*, II (New York, 1892), 172.

criticized Haeckel and others for overlooking Wells. This seemed inexplicable to Jenkins, who claimed that this physician—nearly fifty years before Darwin published the *Origin of Species*—"solved the problem and turned over to thinkers and doers the key to unlock, in a more or less routinary way, the door leading to the sublimity of life, that all inquiring minds might see for themselves." [6]

The obvious retort to this sweeping claim is to say that even if Wells did forge a key to the understanding of evolution, no one used it. There is no evidence that he exerted any direct influence on the evolutionary theories of either his contemporaries or his successors. And this fact might well be cited by historians as justifying their neglect of the man, on the ground that "firsts" which have no apparent connection with subsequent developments are of only antiquarian or patriotic concern.

This generalization would commend itself to most historians, but one qualification may be mentioned in passing. It is a little dangerous to assume that because a given piece of work had no direct influence, it therefore exerted none at all. One of the curious things about Wells' theory is that, while so largely overlooked or forgotten, it was never entirely lost to sight. A nice illustration of this is to be found in the circumstances surrounding Darwin's reference to it. In the "Historical Sketch" to later editions of his *Origin,* the latter quoted Wells and then remarked: "I am indebted to Mr. Rowley of the United States; for having called my attention, through Mr. Brace, to the above passage in Dr. Wells' works." In a subsequent letter to Sir J. D. Hooker, Darwin also remarked: "Talking of the 'Origin' a Yankee has called my attention to a paper attached to Dr. Wells' famous 'Essay on

[6] *Journal American Medical Association,* March 13, 1909, p. 905. See also F. L. Pleadwell, "That Remarkable Philosopher and Physician, Wells of Charleston," *Annals of Medical History,* IV (New York, 1934), 128 ff.

Dew,' . . . in which he applies most distinctly the principle
of Natural Selection to the Races of Man. . . ." [7] From this it
is clearly implied that a certain American not only recalled
Wells' theory as late as 1860, but recognized the similarity to
Darwin's views as soon as the latter's *Origin* appeared. Casual
search has revealed nothing regarding the details of this story.
If the "Mr. Brace" noted was Charles Loring Brace, it is
known that he was much interested in evolution and in touch
with Darwin; [8] but "Mr. Rowley" has not been identified. If
something were known of the latter's familiarity with Wells'
theory, it might throw light on its possible—even if obscure—
influence on the biological thought of the mid-nineteenth
century.

Granting this minor qualification, it remains true that
Wells' influence was slight at best, and that historians—if
they knew of his hypothesis at all—have naturally abandoned
it to the antiquarians. In doing so, however, they have
overlooked a quite different aspect of the matter, which is of
considerable significance. Admitting that Wells' view was
largely lost, *why* was it so lost? Attempted answers to this
question must consider the varied factors which influence the
dissemination of scientific ideas, and here one obviously
emerges on a level of inquiry above that of mere antiquar-
ianism. In a word, Wells affords a striking test case in the
study of what one might term intellectual dynamics. True, it
is a sort of negative case—inertia rather than change is
apparent—but it is not necessarily less revealing for that
reason. [9]

[7] Francis Darwin (ed.), *The Life and Letters of Charles Darwin* (New
York, 1887), p. 225.
[8] See Emma Brace (ed.), *Life of Charles Loring Brace* (New York,
1894), pp. 319 ff.
[9] The analysis which follows relates to what J. D. Bernal (*The Social
Function of Science*, New York, 1939, p. 130) terms the "scientific," as
distinct from the technical and the economic obstacles to the development
of science. For his purpose, he was able to dismiss the "scientific" factors,

The usual explanations given for instances in which a scientist has lacked recognition are (1) he was personally unknown, (2) his work appeared in minor publications, (3) he aroused personal antagonisms, (4) his writing was obscure, (5) his ideas were of no interest to contemporaries—they were "ahead of the times," (6) his thought aroused opposition in terms of various cultural factors making for intellectual inertia.[10] The possible application of each of these to Wells' case may be considered in turn, and then other explanations may be added.

While Wells' personality was such that he had few friends, these few were outstanding men—David Hume, Sir Benjamin Brodie, and others. Moreover, his writings were well known in his own day and were extensively quoted.[11] The particular paper in which he advanced the hypothesis of natural selection was first read in 1813 before the Royal Society. Although this body no longer, at that time, played the role in English science that it once had, it should still have served as a fairly good sounding board. The essay was later printed, in 1818, in a volume also including his "Two Essays: One Upon Single Vision With Two Eyes; The Other on Dew," etc. Both of these latter papers attracted wide attention, and the volume including them and the paper here of concern could scarcely be viewed as in any way obscure. At first glance, then, neither the first nor second explanations noted above would seem applicable to Wells' case.

With reference to the third explanation—the retarding influence of personal antagonisms—there is no question that

---

taking for granted the lag caused by them between first expressions of a new idea and its general acceptance. As "scientific" lag may prove as long or even longer than that due to the other factors, however, it would seem worthy of analysis—even if this has to be done in rather simple or common-sense terms.

[10] Note the analysis of these factors in Bernhard J. Stern, *Social Factors in Medical Progress* (New York, 1927), especially Chapter 1.

[11] Keil, *op. cit.*, p. 791.

Wells did offend his contemporaries, and had no knowledge of "how to win friends and influence people." But since most of his writings were, despite this, well regarded, there is no reason to hold that here was a factor applicable to only a particular paper.

It is equally difficult to believe that Wells' thought in relation to evolution was obscure to his contemporaries. While nothing approaching the later popular interest in the subject had then appeared, it is well known that a considerable number of thinkers had given it or were giving it serious consideration at the time that the London physician spoke and published. Addressed to such men, his essay should have offered no difficulties. Indeed, its clarity and simplicity are such that it is hard to see why it should not have been intelligible to any educated reader. Note, for example, such passages as the following:

> . . . amongst men, as well as among other animals, varieties of a greater or less magnitude are constantly occurring. In a civilized country . . . those varieties, for the most part, quickly disappear, from the intermarriages of different families. . . . In districts, however, of very small extent, and having little intercourse with other countries, an accidental difference in the appearance of the inhabitants will often descend to their late posterity. . . . Again, those attend to the improvement of domestic animals, when they find individuals possessing . . . the qualities they desire, couple a male and female of these together, then take the best of their offering as a new stock, and in this way proceed till they approach as near the point in view as the nature of things will permit. *But, what is here done by art, seems to be done with equal efficacy, though more slowly, by nature, in the formation of varieties of mankind, fitted for the country which they inhabit.*[12] Of the accidental varieties of man, which would occur among the first few and scattered

[12] Italics my own.

inhabitants of . . . Africa, some would be better fitted than the others to bear the diseases of the country. This race would consequently multiply, while the others would decrease, not only from their inability to sustain the attacks of disease, but from their incapacity of contending with their more vigorous neighbors.[13]

Here one apparently has, in essence, the theory of the origin of new forms by a natural selection of accidental variations in the struggle for existence, much as Darwin gave it in greater detail a half century later. Short of using words of one syllable, it is hard to see how the statement could have been made more simple and clear. One can hardly claim, then, that obscurity of expression played much part in this story.

A negative finding must also be reported for the possibility that Wells' views on this subject aroused conscious opposition as a matter of cultural inertia. Here his experience was quite the opposite of Darwin's. If any conservative theologian or other critic ever took the trouble to refute Wells, there is no record of it. On the other hand, in so far as Darwin's views were actually spread by controversy, his predecessor enjoyed no such unintentioned support. Hence the truism that it were better to be attacked than to be ignored, does apply to Wells; but this still offers no explanation of why he was so unfortunate in this respect.

It has already been suggested that Wells was "ahead of his time" in the sense that in his day there was as yet no widespread interest in biological evolution. There is no question that the world was "ready" for Darwin as it was not for Wells. The whole development of the idea of progress, coupled with a faith in laissez faire as the most efficient means to this end, had gone much further by 1860 than it had in 1810. The nicety with which the hypothesis of natural selection fitted

[13] *Two Essays,* etc. (London, 1818), pp. 434 ff.

into this milieu was such that its acceptance was probably more due to social than to biological considerations.[14] Zirkle has pointed out, indeed, that Darwinism began and—in relation to general acceptance—ended in sociology. It was thus, in effect, a tributary to biological thinking that became better known than the main stream.[15]

It is not clear whether Wells' work lies in this main stream or not, for the reason that—unlike Darwin—he gave no clues as to the origin of his ideas. He only remarks that these "occurred to me" while considering the contrasts between Negroes and Europeans. Like that of any scientist, his work presumably was the product of both the surrounding culture and of his individual imagination.[16] With regard to the first factor, Zirkle believes his immediate starting point may have been the work of Pritchard in physical anthropology.[17] If so, neither in origin nor in application was there any conscious connection between Wells' reasoning and social phenomena. Had there been such, even the limited development of the ideas of progress and of laissez faire which had been attained by 1813, might have given his thought wider circulation.

Yet even granting this, no explanation is afforded of the simple question: Why did Wells fail to reach even the limited audience of anthropologists and biologists who had long been interested in his problem?

Up to this point it has been assumed that Wells really did

[14] Nordenskiöld, *History of Biology*, pp. 477 ff.

[15] "Natural Selection Before the 'Origin of Species'," *Proceedings* American Philosophical Society, lxxxiv (1941), pp. 72, 73. For the American story in particular, see Richard Hofstadter, *Social Darwinism in American Thought 1860–1915*, Philadelphia, 1944, a volume in the Beveridge Memorial series of the American Historical Association.

[16] See the analysis of the relative roles of cultural environment and individual "imagination" in A. L. Porterfield, *Creative Factors in Scientific Research*, etc. (Durham, North Carolina, 1941), pp. 39 ff., 88 ff.

[17] Pritchard's main work dealt with just the problems in which Wells was interested and appeared in English in 1813—the year in which the latter read his paper relating to evolution, Zirkle, *op. cit.*, pp. 104 ff.

anticipate Darwin. The latter's own statement, quoted above, has usually been viewed as a generous recognition of the fact. But reading further in this statement, one encounters qualifications. Wells, remarks Darwin, "applies it [the theory of natural selection] only to the races of man and to certain characters alone." [18] This would suggest that the earlier writer had no conception of the wider applications of the hypothesis. Accepting the same view, a recent critic remarks that Wells' "partial anticipation" was not at all the same thing as a "complete development" of the theory.[19] In so far as this is true, it might explain to some degree the lack of interest in the essay of 1813.

To what extent then did this paper really anticipate Darwin? Obviously, it failed to do so in terms of experimentation, or in the massing of any other evidence. Wells collected no data and apparently referred only to such illustrations as occurred to him in passing. And here one can see that Darwin was likely to receive more attention, for the simple reason that he "backed up" his ideas with a wide range of evidence.

To the essential question concerning the completeness of Wells' theory, however, the answer is clear. He put together two hitherto isolated ideas which had long been familiar to biologists—"natural selection" and the "origin of species"—in an essentially new combination.[20] And it was just this combination which constituted the essence of Darwin's later hypothesis. Whatever the cultural background, Wells' reasoning therefore affords a striking example of the role of creative imagination in scientific work. His performance appears the

[18] "Historical Sketch," in *The Origin of Species* (5th ed., New York, 1871), p. 10.

[19] Keil, "Dr. William Charles Wells," etc. *Bulletin of the Institute of the History of Medicine,* iv, 803, footnote. Osborn also implied that Wells failed to see the wider applications; *From the Greeks to Darwin,* p. 221.

[20] Pritchard had hovered on the brink of this achievement but never quite "made it"; Zirkle, *op. cit.,* pp. 104 ff.

more remarkable for the fact that no one else advanced the completed theory, so far as is known, for a decade or more thereafter. This then was no case of "multiple discovery," i.e., of the culture of a given moment irresistibly producing a particular idea.

But what of the qualifications in Darwin's statement? He was, strictly speaking, correct in saying that Wells applied his view "only to the races of mankind." Note again the latter's declaration that:

> . . . what is here done by art, [*re* domestic animal breeding] seems to be done, with equal efficiency, though more slowly, by nature, in the formation of *varieties of mankind.*[21]

Wells might have easily substituted for the last word here the term "animals." It would have followed quite logically from the preceding reference to animal breeding and one almost wishes he could have guided the pen at this point! But the fact remains that the theory was specifically applied only to "varieties of mankind." Whether the author did so because he did not see the applicability to animal forms, or whether he specified mankind only because that was the concern of the moment,[22] is a nice question. The answer depends upon one's interpretation of the context.

The view here taken is that Wells plainly envisaged the theory as applicable to animal forms, but was interested only in its relationship to his immediate problem.[23] Note the

[21] Italics my own.

[22] Wells was trying to account for changes in the colors of races. In his period there was considerable interest in accounting for the origin of racial variations; indeed he was not the only American interested in the problem. It was not until later that anthropologists turned to merely descriptive studies; see M. F. Ashley Montagu, "The Genetical Theory of Race, and Anthropological Method," *American Anthropologist,* xliv (1942), 369.

[23] See original statement to this effect in "William Charles Wells," *Dictionary of American Biography,* xix (1936), 645.

phrasing: "But amongst men, *as well as among other animals,*[24] varieties . . . are constantly occurring." He here takes for granted that variations appear throughout the zoölogical realm, but is not primarily concerned with them. Again, in noting that artificial circumstances of civilization may inhibit variation in races, he points out that animal species also may be held constant by artificial control even in a changed environment.[25] The implication is clear that, in the absence of such artificial control, animals would likewise change through natural selection. Reaching the same conclusion, Zirkle observed several years ago that Wells "obviously understood its [the theory's] wider application." [26]

Darwin, moreover, was mistaken in his second qualifying assertion, i.e., that Wells applied his thesis only to "certain characters" of races. Consider again Wells' statement that:

> Of the accidental varieties of man . . . some would be better fitted than the others to bear the diseases of the country. This race would consequently multiply, while the others would decrease, not only from their inability to sustain the attacks of disease, but from their incapacity of contending with their more vigorous neighbors.

This plainly declares that the survival of the race as such, and not merely of particular "characters" thereof, was to be explained by natural selection. It is of interest to medical historians to note, in passing, that the Anglo-American physician here refers to the role of disease in natural selection —a reference which may be plausibly ascribed to his medical background. Here he suggested a major aspect of the struggle

[24] Italics my own.
[25] *Two Essays*, etc., p. 437. Since writing the above I have noted that Kofoid "An American Pioneer," etc., *Scientific Monthly*, LVII (1943), 78, stresses these same two passages.
[26] *Op. cit.*, p. 106.

for survival which Darwin subsequently overlooked or minimized.[27]

One therefore concludes that Darwin was not so careful in
his reference to Wells as he seems usually to have been in
acknowledging predecessors. Anyone reading his "Historical
Sketch" would assume that Wells had no inkling of the
application of his theory to animals in general, and that even
in relation to mankind he saw no explanation of the evolution
of races as such. This statement of Wells' position, far from
constituting "fullest recognition," [28] was really a quite inadequate evaluation.

Had Darwin, after remarking that Wells "applied" his
theory only to human races, added that nevertheless this
application involved a realization of wider meanings, he
would then have reported the whole story. Or had he
declared, more cautiously, that Wells displayed no realization
of the *significance* of applications to zoölogy in general, he
would have been on sounder ground. As already observed,
Wells suggested such applications quite incidentally and
showed no great interest therein. In other words, he formulated the major aspects of Darwin's later thesis and implied
that it was pertinent to zoölogy in general, but made no
explicit statement to that effect.

Worse than this, Wells did not seem to realize the
significance of his ideas even in relation to their limited,
specific applications. Twice, in the course of the essay, he
practically apologizes to the reader for bothering him with

---

[27] At least, it is largely overlooked in the *Origin*, where competition with
the same or similar species, climatic influences, etc., are stressed as the
main dangers faced in the struggle for survival. These factors, of course,
might be broken down in terms of disease, but Darwin rarely does this.

[28] Kofoid uses this phrase, *op. cit.*, p. 78. It should be added, however,
that Darwin later wrote as though recognizing Wells' application of the
theory to races as a whole. See the quotation in Osborn's *From the Greeks
to Darwin*, p. 222.

these speculations. Thus, in introducing the subject, Wells remarks:

> On considering the difference of colour between Europeans and Africans, a view has occurred to me of this subject, which has not been given by any author, whose works have fallen into my hands. I shall, therefore, *venture* to mention it here, *though at the hazard of its being thought rather fanciful than just.*

Again, at the conclusion, he remarks:

> . . . I forbear *trespassing* any longer upon the time of the reader, *in discussing a subject which admits only of conjectural reasoning.*[29]

The half-apologetic tone here is obvious enough. It is in marked contrast to the earnestness and conviction with which Darwin later presented his own views. Whether Wells' attitude was due to some excessive modesty, or to a lack of confidence, is a matter of interpretation. In any case, he not only presented his theory quite incidentally but also in a manner not at all calculated to inspire confidence in others.[30]

The incidental and uncertain manner in which Wells advanced what might have been his major contribution, is further illustrated in his failure to view it as worthy of an independent essay. His ideas were buried in a paper with the unpromising title: "An account of a Female of the White Race of Mankind, Part of Whose Skin Resembles that of a Negro; with Some Observations on the Causes of the Differences in Colour and Form Between the White and Negro Races of Men." The volume in which this was included was

[29] *Two Essays*, etc., pp. 432, 439. Italics my own.
[30] Professor Philip P. Calvert has called my attention to the fact that Radle suggests a similar comparison between Lamark and Darwin, though this may be a matter of opinion; *The History of Biological Theories*, p. 271.

well known, as has been noted, but readers of the famous "Two Essays" probably were not attracted by the title appended thereto. One can readily imagine that students of biological evolution, seeking references, would pass this by.[31]

The manner in which Wells presented his potentially profound contribution may therefore be viewed as explaining much of the indifference with which it was received. The world was not entirely ready for it, as has been noted, but there was no lack of individual thinkers who might have been impressed had the matter been called to their attention with the emphasis and conviction which we now see it deserved. Both Wells' achievement, and his failure to disseminate it, are therefore to be explained as much in terms of his individual psychology as in relation to his cultural environment. The moral would seem to be that scientists, like others, should take themselves seriously.

[31] Kofoid, *op cit.*, p. 78, notes the analogous obscurity of Pattrick Matthew's title "Naval Timber and Arboriculture" (London, 1831), which also concealed a presentation of the Darwinian theory. Matthews, however, was fully recognized by Darwin.

HISTORIOGRAPHY

XIV

Medical Sources
and the Social Historian [1]

It is a truism that limitations are set upon historical research by the nature of the sources available. The fact that certain materials necessary to the study of European history are inaccessible to the American students has doubtless prevented some studies in that field. It is not so generally recognized that materials are rendered just as inaccessible by habits of mind as by great distances. Indeed mental barriers usually prove more difficult to surmount than the merely geographical ones. Newspapers were long stacked in divers places, for example, before John Bach McMaster first thought of using them in the preparation of his studies in American history. Since the files reposed in newspaper offices or in private homes, to which historians were not accustomed to go, the papers were practically inaccessible to the profession.

This situation was unfortunate, not only because various facts escaped the historian, but because new vistas in historiography likewise eluded him. When McMaster was asked how he happened to include the social data for which his history was famous, he replied that he simply "put in what was in the papers." If his recollection was correct, it was a fortunate

[1] Reprinted from *The American Historical Review*, Vol. XLI, No. 3, April, 1936—by permission.

selection of a new type of source, rather than any preconceived theory, which led him to write the "new history."

Since the appearance of the first volume of the *History of the People of the United States,* there has been some further extension in the range of sources frequently employed by historians. It is interesting to recall that while McMaster was examining the newspaper files, his colleague, Professor Cheyney, was extending his research into the more general literary sources. Cheyney decided, writes Professor Conyers Read:

> long before the great mass of us . . . that the arts, and particularly literature, constituted the largest source of material for history in the broad sense, and he made extensive use of them while most of us were limiting our attention to the State Papers, just as though there were not more of Tudor England in Shakespeare than in all the documents combined.[2]

In this manner, one type of source material after another has come within the range of historical investigations. Today historians are justly proud of their catholicity in this respect. A useful chain has been created, in which more varied sources have suggested wider interests, and the latter in turn have promoted a search for still other sources. The need of such a chain of suggestion becomes at once apparent when the work of general historians is contrasted with that of those devoted to such specialized subjects as the history of medicine, of architecture, or of engineering. The tendency among the latter, at least until very recently, has been to consult only the technical literature in their respective fields.

As if in deference to such specialists, the one type of

[2] "Edward Potts Cheyney: As a Writer," in William E. Lingelbach, ed., *Portrait of an Historian* (Philadelphia, 1935), p. 22.

material still neglected by general historians is the technical literature. This is notably true in the case of the history of science. Materials reposing only a few yards from the historian's office, are for all practical purposes ten thousand miles away, simply because they are within buildings occupied by the professional schools. Most historians are not accustomed to pursue their researches in these institutions. To the extent that the scholar's training does not equip him to use technical materials, he is in a sense justified in this attitude—although a new training program is obviously indicated in this connection.[3] Pending the acquisition of such training, there is still considerable material in technical sources which is intelligible to any capable historian.

It may be that the neglect of scientific literature is due not so much to deference as to indifference. As historians become interested in the cultural significance of science—which certainly looms so large on the intellectual horizon that it can no longer be minimized—they will doubtless employ technical sources. Harvey's papers are just as accessible as Cromwell's—those of Benjamin Rush just as readable as the outpourings of his friend Thomas Jefferson. Much technical literature will doubtless come into its own in this fashion, as

[3] A fact formally recognized in the report of a recent committee on the planning of research, submitted to the American Historical Association (*Historical Scholarship in America,* New York, 1932, p. 31). Such training will tend to integrate the work of general historians with that of those working in special fields. In so far as the process is already under way, it is being approached from the other end as well; that is, such specialists as the medical historians are beginning to be trained in general history, and to use general historical sources. The most promising training program of this sort, in the United States, is that of the Institute of Medical History at the Johns Hopkins University. For a current example of the use of general sources by a medical historian, see Sanford V. Larkey, M. D., "Public Health in Tudor England," *Am. Jour. of Pub. Health,* xxiv, 1099 ff. (New York, 1934). Such medical historians as Arturo Castiglioni, Paul Diepgen, and Henry E. Sigerist are much interested, at the present time, in integrating medical history with social and cultural developments.

the story of science assumes the place it should have in the synthesis which is general history.

The point to be stressed here, however, is not this inevitable recognition of the history of science. It is rather the fact that scientific sources are pertinent to those phases of history already included in all general narratives, for the actual development of certain sciences possesses social implications of the first order. In no case is this more true than in the history of the vital and far-reaching medical sciences.

There is, to begin with, the history of disease. It is scarcely necessary to labor the point of its social significance. Nor is it necessary, in making this point, to subscribe to the extreme view that whole civilizations waxed and waned simply because of disease variations. What must be recognized is that the history of certain regions has inevitably been conditioned by the diseases obtaining therein. Historians always realized this in the case of great epidemics, and medical historians encouraged them here by emphasizing the story of such disasters. It is easier to find records of a sudden "visitation" than it is to trace obscure, endemic conditions; and once written, the former makes more spectacular reading. Hence the universal attention accorded "the Black Death." Hence also the neglect of contemporary endemic diseases, which in the long run were more fatal and perhaps equally significant in their social consequences.[4]

In Angelo Celli's recently published *History of Malaria in the Roman Campagna,* there is at last made available a great mass of historical evidence demonstrating a direct correlation between malaria and decadence in that region—a correlation that assumes obvious significance as one looks back across the centuries. In England and in the United States there are as yet available only fragmentary data and plausible hypotheses

[4] Mazÿck P. Ravenel, "Endemic Diseases vs. Acute Epidemics," *Am. Jour. of Pub. Health,* x (1920), 761 ff.

concerning the historic role of endemic disease. It is inconceivable, however, that so insidious and deadly an enemy as tuberculosis did not play its part in nineteenth-century England; or that malaria, pellagra, and hookworm infection have exerted no influence in America. The latter ills may well account for some of the backwardness of certain Southern sections, and for the so-called "laziness" of certain Southern peoples.

The sources for this phase of English and of American social history lie buried in various places, but are chiefly available in the medical literature. Not much secondary material is to be found, save in brief introductions to books on particular diseases. The standard works of Hirsch and Creighton [5] relate primarily to epidemics; and the pioneer historical studies of American diseases were of the same character. Thus the versatile Noah Webster wrote voluminously of our native epidemics, the accounts of which he based upon extensive "researches among revolving planets, blazing comets, [and] exploding volcanoes." [6] He made some interesting observations in spite of his astrological leanings, and it is the writer's private opinion that when he turned to lexicography, he was a good epidemiologist "gone wrong."

Even before Webster wrote, Lionel Chalmers had published his essay on the diseases of South Carolina (1776); and William Currie had brought out the first American attempt at medical geography; that is, his *Historical Account of the Climates and Diseases of the United States of America,* published at Philadelphia in 1792. It is interesting to observe, in passing, that this was the same year in which appeared the

[5] August Hirsch, *Handbook of Geographical and Historical Pathology,* tr. by Charles Creighton (London, 1883–1886); Charles Creighton, *History of Epidemics in Britain* (Cambridge, 1891–1894).

[6] *Epidemic and Pestilential Diseases* (2 vols., Hartford, 1799). The phrase is from William Currie, *A Sketch of the Rise and Progress of the Yellow Fever* (Philadelphia, 1800), p. 47.

first volume of L. L. Finke's treatise, which is usually considered the first formal work on medical geography.[7] About a decade later (1801) there appeared, at Charleston, what was probably the first serious attempt in medical historiography published in this country. This was David Ramsay's *Review of the Improvements, Progress, and State of Medicine in the XVIIIth Century,* which included a narrative of the Charleston epidemics of that period.[8] Currie later published two other books on the history and geography of American diseases; the second of which—*A View of the Diseases Most Prevalent in the United States of America* (Philadelphia, 1811)—was the best thing of its kind for this country. The dramatic essays of Benjamin Rush on the Philadelphia fevers may also be recalled.

Endemic diseases received some attention in Currie's works; but the first strictly historical study along this line, in the United States, seems to have been the work of no less a luminary than Oliver Wendell Holmes. Holmes was much concerned, as a young man, lest the records of New England diseases be entirely lost. He went over early accounts of malaria page by page—omitting, he declared, only "some few ecclesiastical papers . . . of Cotton Mather, which being more likely to cause a fever than to mention one, I left to some future investigator." His "Dissertation of Intermittent Fever in New England" won the Boylston prize in 1838, but has long since been largely forgotten.[9]

[7] Leonhard Ludwig Finke, *Versuch einer allgemeinen medizinisch-praktischen Geographie* (3 vols., Leipzig, 1792–1795).

[8] See pp. 35 ff. This is a most interesting essay, and is typical of the period. Present readers may be surprised to find that eighteenth-century writers were just as optimistic about "the triumphs of modern medicine" as anyone is today.

[9] Published in the *Boylston Prize Dissertations* (Boston, 1838), pp. 1 ff.

While a well-considered historical paper of this sort was exceptional [10]—and indeed still is—there was no lack of primary comment in the medical literature on malaria and various other endemic diseases. Professional journals and the transactions of professional societies in all parts of the country were replete, during the first half of the nineteenth century, with accounts of the usual "fevers," [11] and special regions reported in addition on such diseases as were more or less peculiar to them. Western physicians, for example, had much to say of "milk sickness"; while Southern doctors expressed concern over the mysterious *cachexia africana* that devastated the plantations of Louisiana and of the West Indies.

The unsatisfactory nosography of the period renders the use of these reports difficult, since disease classification still rested, as late as 1860, on a symptom-complex or at best on a pathological basis. There has, in consequence, been some disagreement as to what diseases were primarily involved in given instances, particularly during the earlier periods. Holmes in writing of early New England, and contemporary historians describing seventeenth-century Virginia, have agreed that malaria was the chief bane of the founding fathers.[12] Heagerty, on the other hand, believes that scurvy was the main cause of early sickness in Virginia; while Blanton has recently ascribed this tragedy to dysentery and to

[10] It is interesting to note that Holmes was trained in Louis's seminar at Paris, and that the seminar method was introduced in the Boston "Society for Medical Improvement" by Louis's American pupils at this time. This was about a half century before it entered, through German influence, into general historical training in this country.

[11] See, for example, the presidential address of Alexander Coventry, to the New York State Medical Society in 1824 (*Transactions,* I, 257 ff.) in which he recited the tragic history of the fevers in the Seneca Lake country.

[12] See Thomas Jefferson Wertenbaker, *Virginia under the Stuarts* (Princeton, 1922), p. 115; and the same author's *The First Americans* (New York, 1929), pp. 178 ff.

typhoid.[13] Smallpox was not involved in the general fevers, since it was commonly recognized as a distinct disorder.

No doubt typhoid, dysentery, and malaria were all involved, in varying degrees, in the "autumnal fevers" of early settlements; and occasionally dengue or other infectious diseases were present. Respiratory infections certainly constituted the greater part of the "winter fevers"; and scurvy or other malnutrition diseases must have prevailed whenever diets were seriously restricted. Keeping such generalizations in mind, and making allowance for variations in time and place, it is by no means impossible to interpret the early reports on disease. The historian who does interpret them will be rewarded not only by the knowledge of disease history in itself, but by what is of more direct concern to him—new light on social conditions in general. No one can read the endless comments on "fevers" and "fluxes" in new settlements without suspecting that the heroic tradition of the robust frontiersman is a misleading one. The "rugged individualists" of the backwoods were not so rugged after all.

As Garrison and others have pointed out—and indeed as Holmes observed a century ago—the frontier was at first a healthy region. This was the sylvan paradise stage, familiar only to explorers, to fur traders, and to settlers during the first year or so of settlement. Permanent occupation reversed the situation in tragic fashion, since it was attended by a devastating development of the diseases noted. Later, as the frontier-farming stage merged gradually into the humdrum regime of established settlement, the fevers as gradually declined. The rapidity of the process varied widely; such factors as climate, the particular diseases involved, and the distinction between rural and urban conditions all played their part. Yet the

---

[13] John J. Heagerty, *Four Centuries of Medical History in Canada* (Toronto, 1928), I, 7 ff.; Wyndham H. Blanton, *Medicine in Virginia in the Seventeenth Century* (Richmond, 1930), pp. 50 ff.

general pattern is the same, whether one considers the first settlement at Charleston late in the seventeenth century, the migration into the Genesee country at the end of the eighteenth century, or the late coming of the "forty-niners" to California.[14] One could almost define the different stages of settlement in terms of their dominant diseases, as well as by the characteristics more usually noted. It may be added, in passing, that perhaps the earliest published description of these stages, later elaborated in the Turner thesis, is to be found in the essays of the physician Benjamin Rush.[15]

In the more comprehensive writings of another great physician, Daniel Drake, is evidence of the persistence of frontier types of disease for a considerable period and over large areas. This evidence is assembled in the most impressive of all American works on medical geography—Drake's classic volumes on the diseases of the Mississippi Valley.[16] The author traveled all over the great valley for many years, taking careful notes on its climate, flora, fauna, ethnography, and the prevailing diseases. Garrison is convinced that nothing comparable had appeared since the Hippocratic writings. No work of so comprehensive a character can fail to have some value for the social historian.

The reason for this is obvious enough. The physician who reports disease on a social scale almost necessarily relates it to environment. The living conditions associated with a given type of illness are likely to possess causal significance, and must be described along with the symptoms. For the same

[14] St. Julien Ravenel Childs, "Health and Disease in the Early History of South Carolina" (MS. thesis, George Washington University, 1931), pp. 24 ff.; Alexander Coventry, N.Y. State Med. Soc., *Trans.*, I, 257 ff. (1824); E. O. Essig, *A History of Entomology* (New York, 1931), p. 210.

[15] In his papers on Pennsylvania, published in *Essays, Literary, Moral, & Philosophical* (Philadelphia, 1798), pp. 213 ff., 226 ff.

[16] *A Systematic Treatise . . . on the Principal Diseases of the Interior Valley of North America* (Cincinnati, 1850).

reason, a doctor wishing to eradicate a given endemic condition may find it desirable to investigate and to condemn
related social circumstances. So it was that certain physicians
became social reformers, and their writings took on something
of the character of social surveys.

With the advent of the early industrial revolution in
England, for example, physicians were in the van of those
who protested against the dangers of overcrowded and unsanitary slums. An early picture of such conditions can be found
in the first works on medical police—notably in such a study
as Roberton's, which was published in Edinburgh in 1808–
1809.[17] Less formal, but quite interesting are the accounts
given in the medical essays of private practitioners. One of the
best examples is in the "medical histories" of Dr. John Ferriar
of Manchester, written late in the eighteenth century.[18] He
belonged to the famous "Manchester group" of socially
minded physicians which, among other things, did something
to start Robert Owen on his career of amelioration. Ferriar
was not only able to report on the living conditions of the
poor, but he was in a position to do so more intelligently than
were most other observers.

This critical point deserves emphasis. The value of medical
evidence lies not simply in the fact that it is so much more
evidence, but rather in that it may afford the most significant
information available. Because of both the intimate and the
continuous character of his contacts with the poor, the doctor
was more likely to understand their situation than were other
local observers who came into casual association with them. In
like manner, the doctor was—other things being equal—a
more reliable reporter than the traveler who observed only in
passing. This means that the medical literature, relatively

[17] John Roberton, *Medical Police*, etc.
[18] *Medical Histories and Reflections* (London, 1810–1813), ii, 213 ff.

unknown to social historians, affords at times more trustworthy evidence than does the travel literature so religiously consulted by them.

A striking illustration of this is afforded by the history of that truly "peculiar institution," American Negro slavery. It will be recalled that much of the controversy concerning slavery centered about one obvious and basic question. Were or were not the slaves ill treated? Testimony was taken from planters on the one hand, and from English or Northern travelers on the other. Now the former knew slavery well enough, but were naturally biased by their vested interests therein. Some of the travelers were disqualified as observers by just the opposite bias, for they saw the Southern scene obscurely through the glass of abolitionist sentiment.

Of all critics, the Southern physician was perhaps in the best position to report on the physical and moral treatment of the slaves. When he stated, as he sometimes did, that Negroes were overworked and underfed, he can hardly be suspected of antislavery bias since he was the friend of the planter who employed him. As a matter of fact, he usually approved of the institution. Coming into frequent contact with human bondage under the most intimate circumstances, he was in a position to understand it as few travelers could hope to do. On the other hand, his vested interest in the institution was rarely so direct or so great as was that of the planters.

Yet of all sources, it is this relatively reliable professional testimony which is alone neglected by the historians of slavery. It is a rare treatise, for example, which does not cite Frederick Law Olmsted—a Connecticut Yankee at King Cotton's court, a traveler who, having given up farming at home, devoted several long trips to telling the South how to improve its own agriculture. And it is an equally rare study which cites the medical evidence.

This is not to be explained by any lack of material. The

personal comments of physicians in their correspondence are, to be sure, rather inaccessible, since many volumes containing the papers of Southern politicians have been published for every one pertaining to physicians.[19] The evidence is again found chiefly in the medical journals, and in the transactions of medical societies. Some of this related primarily to demography; as did Lemuel Shattuck's important article in the *American Journal of the Medical Sciences,* in which he called attention to an interesting phenomenon, the marked decline of the Negro population in Boston during the eighteenth century.[20]

Writing in the same period, Josiah Nott compared the Negro mortality rates of the chief Eastern seaports during the first half of the nineteenth century. He contrasted the relatively high death rates for free Negroes in Northern cities with the relatively low rates for slaves in the Southern towns. Conscious that the difference here might be ascribed to the influence of climate—since Negroes were supposed to succumb in direct proportion to their distance from ancestral homes—Nott then compared the two groups within the one border city of Baltimore. He found that here, within the same climatic area, free Negroes still perished more frequently than did their brethren in bondage.[21] The physician therefore implied that emancipation would be followed by increasing Negro mortality—the very consequence which actually followed abolition in 1865. Unfortunately, neither abolitionists

[19] It may be remarked, incidentally, that there is a real opportunity here to present to the reading public the correspondence or memoirs of a learned profession, in addition to the many collections now available for political leaders. Those who have read the professional memoirs which have occasionally appeared—for example, the autobiography of Marion Sims—will recall how fascinating these can be.

[20] "On the Vital Statistics of Boston," N. S., i, 371, 377 (Philadelphia, 1841).

[21] "Health and Longevity of the Southern Seaports," *Southern Journal of Medicine and Pharmacy,* ii, 138 (Charleston, 1847).

nor politicians read the medical journals in the days "before the War."

Less abstract commentaries on Negroes and slavery are found in articles relating to the diseases, the hygiene, and the general care of plantation slaves. The *Southern Medical Reports*—a promising journal in which Sir William Osler was later to discover his "Alabama student"—contained specific criticism of the treatment of slaves amid some general praise of the institution. Thomas Affleck of Mississippi, a lay contributor writing on plantation hygiene, reported that Negro diet was deficient in vegetables, and that the pneumonia common in the cabins in winter was "greatly aggravated by the unskilful treatment of the overseers." His comment on the care of Negro children was in sharp contrast to the pleasant traditions that have come down to us by word of mouth in the better families. The slave quarters "are often badly located," he observed, the "children [are] allowed to be filthy; are suckled hurriedly, whilst the mother is overheated"; and "a vast proportion die under nine or ten days, from the most unskilful management of negro midwives." [22]

Another somber aspect of slavery was emphasized by Dr. Pendleton, when he noted the frequency of abortion among Negro women. "All country practitioners," he observed, "are aware of the frequent complaints of planters upon this subject." There were four times as many abortions and miscarriages, in proportion to population, among the Negroes as among the whites. The planters were convinced, according to Pendleton, that the slaves resorted to the use of emmenagogues, but he himself was uncertain on this point. [23] It may be

[22] "On the Hygiene of Cotton Plantations and the Management of Negro Slaves," *Southern Med. Repts.*, II, 432 ff. (New Orleans, 1850). The journal appeared only for this and the preceding year.

[23] E. M. Pendleton, "On the Susceptibility of the Caucasian and African Races to the Different Classes of Disease," *ibid.*, I, 338.

that there is material here for a hitherto unrecognized and somewhat bizarre chapter in the history of birth control in the United States.

The probable persistence of malnutrition diseases among Negroes in the Lower South, long after the days of early settlement, also suggests an unhappy aspect of slave life. The evidence here, like all of that pertaining to the history of disease, is somewhat uncertain and is open to interpretation. It is not absolutely certain that the Negroes suffered from malnutrition—or, if they did, that poor whites did not also suffer in the same degree. It is suggestive, however, that the medical literature reported a serious disease peculiar to Negroes in the West Indies and in the Gulf region in the United States—a disease commonly known, after 1800, by the none too illuminating name of *cachexia africana*. The symptoms were complicated and numerous—including dirt-eating, anemia, edema, melancholy, and heart failure. The progress of the disease was moderately rapid and it was often fatal.

Now that many diseases can be classified on a causal basis, it is easy to see that there was some hookworm infection involved. A study of the earlier French and British literature, as well as the American, leads to the view that serious malnutrition diseases were also present in this typically confused "clinical picture." [24] The relatively rapid and fatal character of the disorder was not typical of hookworm infection; certain symptoms suggest pellagra, and it is also

[24] [J. B.] Dazille, *Observations sur les Maladies des Nègres* (Paris, 1792), I, 342 ff.; Benjamin Rush, "An account of the diseases peculiar to the negroes in the West-Indies, and which are produced by their slavery," *American Museum*, IV, 81 f. (Philadelphia, 1788); John Hunter, *Observations on the Diseases of the Army in Jamaica* (3d ed., London, 1808), pp. 248 ff.; W. M. Carpenter, "Observations on the Cachexia Africana," *New Orleans Medical Journal*, I, 146–168 (1844); F. W. Craigin, "Observations on Cachexia Africana or Dirt-Eating," *Am. Jour. of the Med. Sciences*, XVII, 356 ff. (1836); J. B. Duncan, "On the . . . Diseases of the Parish of St. Mary, La.," *Southern Med. Repts.*, I, 194–195 (1849).

possible that scurvy or beriberi were involved. The distribution of *cachexia africana* coincided with that of large sugar plantations on which Negroes were fed a routine diet of corn bread, salt pork, and molasses; and some physicians reported that the disease was cured by providing a variety of fresh foods. These facts suggest that large gangs of slaves were required, presumably because of the ignorance of their masters, to live upon disease-producing diets.

Professional literature sometimes expressed the political as well as the social spirit of the times. This is well illustrated in Samuel A. Cartwright's contribution to the *Southern Medical Reports* on "The Diseases and Physical Peculiarities of the Negro Race." Cartwright advanced the thesis that the main cause of the whole sectional controversy preceding the Civil War was Northern ignorance concerning matters medical and psychological. For, he declared, "the vulgar error that there is no difference in the negro's organization, physiology and psychology, and that all the apparent difference arises from Southern slavery, is the cause of all those political agitations which are threatening to dissolve our Union. The knowledge to correct this most mischievous error," he added, ". . . is to be found by cultivating comparative anatomy, physiology, history and ethnography." Here is stated a scientific rather than an economic or political cause of the Civil War. The essay formed a part of what might be termed the scientific proslavery movement, which has received less attention than the literary movement directed toward the same end.[25]

It has already been observed that medical men were among the first to protest the evils of industrial towns. They were often leaders in the sanitary reform movement which can be

[25] *Ibid.*, II, 429. There was quite a body of such literature, including sociological, anthropological, and medical writings. Such authors as Fitzhugh, Hundley, Nott, and Van Evrie are already well known in this connection.

traced to the later eighteenth century, but which did not acquire much headway until after 1830. During the next two decades, the major reports on living conditions in industrial slums were prepared by socially minded physicians. Drs. Villermé of Paris, Arnott, Kay, and Smith of London, Griscom of New York, and Virchow of Berlin are perhaps the best examples. Their individual descriptions of living conditions in Paris, in London, in New York, and in Silesia are valuable sources for the social history of the period.[26] But these were transcended by another type of medical literature; namely, the medical survey in which numbers of physicians co-operated to portray the living conditions of a given area, in some cases of an entire nation.

The most important example of this was the famous English Poor Law Board report of 1842, in which a lay sanitarian, Edwin Chadwick, analyzed the local statements submitted by the poor law doctors for every "union" in England. Supplementary data for parts of Scotland were included.[27] Although this report on "the Sanitary Condition of the Labouring Population" was in origin an investigation of the poor law medical system, it afforded in fact a picture of the living conditions of the poorer urban classes throughout Great Britain. None of the other social investigations of the

[26] [Louis René] Villermé, "Mémoire sur la mortalité en France dans la classe aisée et dans la classe indigente," *Mém.*, Académie de médecin (Paris, 1828); and the same author's *Tableau de l'état physique et moral des ouvriers employés dans les manufactures de coton, de laine, et de soie* (2 vols., Paris, 1840); N. Arnott and J. P. Kay, "On the Prevalence of Certain Physical Causes of Fever in the Metropolis," in appendix to the *Fourth Annual Report of the Poor Law Commissioners* (London, 1838); Southwood Smith, "Report on some of the Physical Causes of Sickness and Mortality," etc., *ibid.*; John H. Griscom, *The Sanitary Condition of the Laboring Population of New York* (New York, 1845); Rudolf Virchow, "Mittheilungen über die in Oberschlesienherschende Typhus-Epidemie," *Archiv für pathologische Anatomie* (Berlin, 1848).

[27] *Report . . . on an Enquiry into the Sanitary Condition of the Labouring Population of Great Britain, with Appendices* (London, 1842).

period, such as the studies made in the mines and in the factories, compared with it in scope. If one really wishes to know how the urban masses lived in early Victorian England, this great medical survey is the place *par excellence* in which to find that information.

Similar investigations could hardly be made by physicians in the United States, where there was no Federal medical system. The National Institute of Washington attempted for some years to arrange for a survey, and finally persuaded the American Medical Association to undertake a study of urban conditions. The reports returned by that organization's committee on hygiene, in 1848 and in 1849, contain some of the first critical descriptions of slum conditions in growing American cities.[28] Meanwhile, Lemuel Shattuck directed and drafted (1850) a famous sanitary survey of Massachusetts which threw considerable light on living conditions in that region.[29] No other state, however, was sufficiently progressive to provide for a similar study; and when Dr. John Shaw Billings revived in 1880 the plan for a great national survey, it was defeated by general indifference.[30] Had this study ever been made, it would have afforded a cross-section view of American living conditions comparable to that of English life provided in the *Report* of 1842.

Special surveys, fortunately, comprised but a small part of the literature relating to the public health. As permanent health departments were established in progressive countries —first local or provincial bodies, later national offices as well —they issued regular reports which included no little mate-

---

[28] See the Am. Med. Assoc., *Transactions,* i, 305 ff.; ii, 431 ff. (Philadelphia, 1848, 1849).

[29] *Report on the Sanitary Condition of Massachusetts* (Boston, 1850).

[30] Fielding H. Garrison, "Geomedicine: a Science in Gestation," *Bulletin of the Institute of the History of Medicine,* vol. i, no. 1 p. 5 (Suppl. to the *Bulletin* of the Johns Hopkins Hospital, vol. lii, no. 1 (Baltimore, January, 1933).

rial of social significance. Historians owe a considerable debt
to cholera, in this connection, for it was largely fear of this
disease which prompted the organization and publications of
health departments between 1830 and 1880. Anyone interested in the public health movement per se, naturally must
use these official documents; and they have been consulted
occasionally by general historians. It is only to be mentioned,
in passing, that the American literature includes materials
dating as early as the eighteenth century, and that some quite
extensive publications are available—such as the proceedings
of the important national sanitary conventions of 1857–1860,
and the *Papers* and *Journal* of the American Public Health
Association. General histories of the public health have been
prepared for certain European nations, of which the most
notable is Fischer's recent work on Germany.[31] No such study
has been made for the United States, but a number of able
works relating to the history of special regions or to special
phases of the American story have appeared in recent decades.[32]

---

[31] Alfons Fischer, *Geschichte des deutschen Gesundheitswesens* (2 vols.,
Berlin, 1933). Note also Sir John Simon, *English Sanitary Institutions*
(London, 1890); and Sir Malcolm Morris, *The Story of English Public
Health* (London, 1919). Sir Arthur Newsholme's *International Studies*
(London and Baltimore, 1931) and his work, in collaboration with John
Adams Kingsbury, entitled *Red Medicine: Socialized Health in Soviet
Russia* (New York, 1933), afford detailed information on recent history
throughout Europe.

[32] References are given in the author's "Origins of the Public Health
Movement in the United States," *Annals of Medical History*, N.S., I,
654 ff. (Philadelphia, 1929). The most valuable local history is William
Travis Howard, *Public Health Administration and the Natural History of
Disease in Baltimore, Maryland, 1797–1920* (Washington, 1924). Proba-
bly the best state history is that of Massachusetts, given in George
Chandler Whipple, *State Sanitation* (Cambridge, 1917). An outstanding
study of Federal health work is Robert D. Leigh's, *Federal Health
Administration in the United States* (New York, 1927), which includes
much historical material. Mazÿck P. Ravenel, ed., *A Half Century of
Public Health* (New York, 1921), contains short historical articles which
afford the most comprehensive picture of later American developments.

Works on personal hygiene, as well as on public hygiene, reveal the habits of a people. This is true of the older histories of health, and books on hygiene proper. The first of these histories, in English, is probably that of James Mackenzie (1758); [33] but far more valuable is the encyclopedic work of Sir John Sinclair, published at Edinburgh in 1807.[34] The later work contains, among much other matter, a bibliography listing nearly nineteen hundred items, and an interesting section on the development of sports and games which has much the character of a source for eighteenth-century Britain. To one who does not share the prevailing mania for golf, it is quite encouraging to find therein a lament that the grand old game of Scotland went into a decline during that period. The implication that a similar fate may befall it in twentieth-century America is most encouraging.

Less obvious is another type of literature which is medical in a broad sense of the term. The popular health papers and journals were often ephemeral as individual publications, but were most persistent as a type in this country from about 1830 to the present time. Some are largely worthless, but others— such as the Grahamite papers—at least afford interesting sidelights on the habits and customs of their time, from bathing to birth control.[35]

It is generally recognized, finally, that the history of the medical profession itself represents a significant phase of social and cultural evolution. Excellent work has been done by medical historians, as by Packard and recently by Sigerist,[36]

[33] *The History of Health and the Art of Preserving It* (Edinburgh).

[34] *Code of Health and Longevity* (4 vols., Edinburgh).

[35] E.g., the Boston *Health Journal and Advocate of Physiological Reform* (1840); the New York *Herald of Health,* which had a long run in that city after *ca.* 1850.

[36] Francis R. Packard, *History of Medicine in the United States* (2d ed., 2 vols., New York, 1931); Henry E. Sigerist, *Amerika und die Medizin* (Leipzig, 1933); and the same work, translated by Hildegard Nagel under the title *American Medicine* (New York, 1934).

in tracing the American story; but the subject is a complicated one, and probably merits further study. It includes such phases as the history of professional training and licensing, the related difficulties with quackery and sectarianism, the development of professional ethics, and the now much mooted question of the organization and economics of medical practice.[37] The single topic of the relation of American medicine to the European, affording as it does a specific illustration of the transition of culture across the Atlantic, is worthy of the most careful investigation.

On all these matters, the publications of nearly every local and state medical society, to say nothing of individual essays and regular journals, contain a vast amount of pertinent material. This is not at all technical in character, and occasionally approaches the level of genuine literature. There are few more enlightening essays on the status of American culture, for example, than the reports on American medical literature submitted to the American Medical Association between 1848 and 1852. These essays seem to be little known, apparently because they remain buried in the *Transactions* of the association. It was here that Holmes, voicing that same interest in a national culture which animated Emerson and other contemporaries, deplored the continued colonial dependence of medical authors upon British publications. Most native writers, he declared, were simply putting "English portraits of disease in American frames." [38]

[37] It may be observed that the final report of the "Committee on the Costs of Medical Care" (*Medical Care for the American People*, Chicago, 1932) contains data which will probably prove of great value to the future historian. Dr. Harry H. Moore, who served as director of this study, also contributed a section on "Health and Medical Practice" to President Hoover's report on *Recent Social Trends* (New York, 1933), ii, 1061 ff., which will probably have a similar value.

[38] Am. Med. Assoc., *Trans.*, i, 283–288 (Philadelphia, 1848). I am assuming here that Holmes wrote this report, since he was chairman of the committee on medical literature which submitted it that year. The style also would suggest his authorship.

Even the most technical medical literature is occasionally of some general interest. It may directly reflect the whole intellectual tone of a given period, as does the speculative German work of the *naturphilosophie* era early in the nineteenth century. Or, again, the introductory sections of a technical work may prove suggestive, when the remainder of its pages are quite barren for the general reader. Thus an introductory letter, in a work by Dr. Charles D. Meigs, contains a typically Victorian tribute to the "genteel female" which should prove of passing interest to the historian of feminism. The good doctor solemnly assures his students that woman's "intellectual force is different from that of her master and lord"; and after much more to the same effect, concludes that her place is in the home "except when, like the star of day, she deigns to issue forth to the world, to exhibit her beauty and her grace." [39] All this sweetness and light went to make up a lecture on obstetrics. It would be difficult to find anything sweeter—or lighter, for that matter—in the hearts and flowers literature of the period.

Here and there throughout his pages, Meigs refers to his patients as "the dear little ladies"—a phrase which now appears somewhat incongruous in such a setting. The Victorians could practice a sort of brutal realism, however, for all their sentiment. It was this same influential physician who denied his "dear ladies" the benefit of aseptic procedures, when these were first advocated by the critical Dr. Holmes. The resulting controversy between the Boston anatomist and the Philadelphia obstetrician was one of the most dramatic in the history of American medicine.

It would be easy, it may be observed in conclusion, to exaggerate the value of medical sources in general historiography. The greatest part of this literature is naturally of

[39] "Sexual Peculiarities" (Letter IV), in *Females and Their Diseases* (Philadelphia, 1848), pp. 40 ff.

interest only to medical men. But this affords no reason for overlooking the pertinent material which is there. The necessity for working through many irrelevant pages is by no means peculiar to the use of professional literature. It is the typical experience, as many a distracted searcher knows, of those who struggle through newspaper files. And here one distinct advantage inheres in the use of medical sources. Probably no other materials can be so easily checked and located. We owe this largely to the development of American library technique and bibliographical organization.

Until almost 1880, physicians had available only catalogues for special subjects or for individual authors. But about that year, the U.S.A. Surgeon General's Library began to issue the *Index Medicus* of current publications, and also the first series of its great *Index Catalogue.* The first edition of the latter was completed in 1895, a second in 1916, a third in 1933, and a fourth is under way. No less than forty-eight large volumes have been published to date. The presiding genius in the original preparation of this work was John Shaw Billings, a versatile physician who later became the first director of the New York Public Library.[40] He was ably assisted by Robert Fletcher and by Fielding H. Garrison. Today, the Surgeon General's Library contains nearly a million volumes and probably constitutes the greatest medical library in existence. In the *Catalogue,* a standard reference work the world over, the historian will find the most specific subject as well as author headings, and under each of these both books and a select list of periodical items in all European languages. A considerable percentage of the more important materials listed here will also be found in other large medical libraries.

[40] See Walter F. Willcox, "John Shaw Billings," *Dict. Am. Biog.,* ii, 266 ff.; and, for the full account, Fielding H. Garrison, *John Shaw Billings: a Memoir* (New York, 1915).

The facilities thus afforded for checking medical sources make their use seem relatively simple and final in comparison with the exploitation of ordinary newspapers or correspondence. There have always been individual historians, of course, who used medical materials; and a number of American historians have recently made more general use of these sources.[41] Yet it is still true, that there is no other great corpus of literature which is so little employed by scholars at large.[42] The *Index Catalogue* itself is not mentioned in excellent manuals of historical bibliography, which list with great care practically all other guides available.

It is a fair prediction that once historians become familiar with the great bibliographical tool which Billings developed they will consult the medical sources more frequently and more systematically. The historical needle in the medical haystack is not so hard to find after all, and is sometimes well worth the searching.

[41] Notably Lynn Thorndike and other medievalists interested in the history of European science. A recognition of the value of medical sources for American social history will be found in several of the volumes of the History of American Life series, edited by Dixon R. Fox and Arthur M. Schlesinger. Examples of the intensive use of medical materials are afforded in such recent American biographies as Nathan G. Goodman, *Benjamin Rush* (Philadelphia, 1934); and Courtney Robert Hall, *A Scientist in the Early Republic, Samuel Lotham Mitchill, 1764–1831* (New York, 1934).

[42] Unless it is the legal literature. This is another story.

XV

The Need for Studies
in the History
of American Science *

It is a truism that no factor has been more important, in the evolution of contemporary society, than the natural sciences and their technological applications. In many ways, science has been the most dynamic influence in making our present culture—in both its material and immaterial aspects—so different from that of preceding centuries. The history of the sciences, therefore, deserves emphasis in all accounts of the development of modern civilization.

Unfortunately, there is rarely any such emphasis in general historical narratives. Recent accounts of this nature have usually been written, in the United States, by professional historians. Prior to about 1900, these scholars stressed economic or political themes. Since then they have gradually given more attention to social and cultural developments; but science, in comparison with social movements, literature, and the fine arts, has fared badly even in this so-called "New History." Few professional historians have attempted studies of any given subject like physics or chemistry; and their discussions of science in general have usually been inade-

* Reprinted from *ISIS*, xxxv, Part 1, No. 99 (Winter, 1944). Copyright, 1944, by *The History of Science Society, Inc.*—by permission.

quate. Often these have been too brief, when present at all. A recent and otherwise superior text on "American History since 1914," gives as much as three pages to the work of a single literary figure like Sherwood Anderson, but less than a paragraph to the whole story of pure science in this period. In other cases, the comment fails to convey any real understanding of the problems or trends in the field noted.

The explanation of this is obvious enough. The training of historians continued to be largely political or literary in nature, long after they had transcended political themes and had ceased to be especially concerned with literary skills. Lacking training in science, even those who recognized its significance tended to avoid so unfamiliar a theme. Or, if they felt bound to include it, the discussion was likely to be of a superficial nature. Literature and the fine arts fared better, because here the scholar felt more at home.

The scientist would probably agree with these statements, and—if he were concerned at all—be inclined to blame historians for not having taken the training necessary for the interpretation of technical fields. Yet the historian could just as well blame the scientist. The former can hold that general history is not a subject in itself, but rather a synthesis of all phases of the past. And these specific themes should be handled by specialists. Why have the chemists not prepared more adequate histories of chemistry? If these were available, then professional historians could incorporate the findings in their own narratives. It may be added, incidentally, that the same reply could be made to social scientists, who sometimes bewail the lack of studies in social history by historians. It is the latter who may claim the grievance: why have sociologists not traced the story of the family that historians need for their syntheses?

Once again, the explanation is obvious. The scientist knows his technical field but is usually unfamiliar with historical sources, methods, background, points of view. His writings are apt to be of an antiquarian character and to lack unity, emphasis and coherence—simple as these literary qualities may seem at first glance. Thus, Garrison's *History of Medicine* is so disjointed that it can hardly claim to be a narrative, though it is valuable as a reference work. Even if an individual scientist happens to possess literary skill, his account of a particular field often is not related to the social background. And science can be no more understood out of relation to its total setting than the latter can be without reference to science.

In other words, if a chemist or biologist essays to write the history of his field, he needs historical training, just as a historian who wishes to deal with the same theme requires some degree of technical understanding. There is no need to decide which of these two types employs the best approach— the scientist or the historian. It may be that, in terms of their respective backgrounds, the scientist will be at his best in relatively technical accounts, the professional historian in the broader or more generalized interpretations. But there is work aplenty for both, and cooperation is clearly indicated.

All that has been said applies with especial force to American history. Conversely, more exceptions could be claimed in the case of writings on European history. In the latter sphere, we do have in English such standard works on the sciences as those of Sarton and of Thorndike, and a number of excellent studies of specific fields or periods.

Far different is the situation in American history. Such studies as those mentioned rarely give much heed to the American fringe of European culture. Even "U-S-A-sian" scholars or scientists writing in this field have rarely dealt with the story of their own country. There is, of course, a cumulative literature on the history of American science, but most of this is in the nature of articles, biographies, and collections of short essays. With a very few exceptions, comprehensive studies—similar to the many works on other phases of national development—have never appeared. Where, for example, are treatments of American science as a whole comparable to Kirkland's *History of American Economic Life,* or the *Cambridge History of American Literature?* Or the studies of special sciences, comparable to the innumerable works on special phases of our economic, political, religious, or literary evolution?

It may be that bibliographical checks would reveal a number of works on given sciences which are not well known, for these sometimes turn up unexpectedly. A history of American anthropology was published ten years ago, of all places in Calcutta. But a study that is little known hardly meets the needs here under consideration.

It is easy to see why histories of science have usually ignored national boundaries, whether of this or any other country. Each sovereign state necessarily has its own political, and to some extent its own economic story, but this is not so clear in the case of science. The latter has always maintained international ideals in large degree; and a nationalistic approach to its history might distort both the facts and the whole spirit of true science. It is quite plausible to conclude that American activities should be noted only when these emerged on the level of international significance.

But there is another side to this picture. If the history of scientific work done in this country is ignored, save at the points where it occasionally attracted international attention, much that was significant for the story of the American people is lost. And we certainly wish to trace the cultural development of our people as a whole. In a word, the value of studies in the history of American science is not to be found primarily in contributions to the history of science as such, but rather to the history of the United States.

There is a close parallel here to the current interest in other phases of our national culture; for example, to the history of American literature. Many scholars working in this field feel that their labors are directed toward enriching our knowledge of national life rather than toward a study of art for its own sake. Another parallel may be found in research on the history of American religion. Religious ideals are presumably international in nature and the great landmarks in religious history have not graced the American horizon; yet no one doubts the importance of integrating American religious history with other phases of national development.

Once it is agreed that the study of the history of science within any particular country is essential to the larger story of that country, further observations may be submitted which guard against the limitations of the nationalistic approach. First, writers on American—or British, or French—science should consciously guard against nationalistic prejudice. Second, they should "keep an eye out" for evidence in their respective territories of any phenomena of international significance that may hitherto have been overlooked. These may occasionally relate to a particular person, idea, or discovery. In the case of American science, to be specific, more adequate accounts might do something to achieve greater recognition abroad. To the extent that American work may have been discounted because of disdain for a colonial culture, such recognition may at times be really deserved. There have been individual Americans like Beaumont or Willard Gibbs, who were more appreciated in Europe than at home; but by and large, Europeans know as little of our scientific as of other phases of our national past. I once enjoyed a discussion with an able German medical historian who could not recall a single American physician prior to Osler, although he was able to check in his library on Benjamin Rush, when that gentleman was mentioned. It was presumably to remedy this situation that Sigerist published at Leipzig, during the 1930's, his *Amerika und die Medizin;* but such interpretive efforts in Europe have been few and far between.

In other cases, a knowledge of American experience might throw new light on that of the "old countries"—by way of contrast. Thus an understanding of the handicaps suffered by scientists here because of a lack of certain attitudes or institutions may lead to new evaluations of the latter as these did actually develop overseas. In these ways, a properly conducted study of national history may, as a sort of by-product, improve our understanding of even the international record.

In reviewing the actual history of American science, one is often struck by the lag in research in this country as compared with the record of western Europe. This can hardly be explained by the lack of sufficient population and wealth to support pure science in a new land, since American resources in this respect were more than adequate a century ago. No doubt various factors explain the contrast, but one major influence seems to have been the prevailing attitude of the American people towards science and scholarship as such. Research lacked the prestige in this country that was accorded it in most European states, and consequently also lacked until recently the essential support of individuals, corporations, or governments. It is a question whether, even down to the present War, pure science—or pure scholarship for that matter—received the general respect in the U.S.A. that has long been obvious in such countries as Germany and Russia.

Here the practical inventor like Edison was widely respected, while Willard Gibbs was largely ignored.

This American attitude, whatever its historical explanations, is deeply embedded in our national tradition and even in our contemporary culture. It was illustrated, until recently, by contrasting public attitudes toward the "professor" in Germany and in the United States. It is also reflected in the very lack of interest in the history of science in this country, which is the subject of the present statement.

Conversely, it follows that *one way to overcome American indifference to research is to give more attention to its history.* As special studies on the history of American science appear, something of their contents will percolate into college texts on our national story, and from these both facts and viewpoints may eventually reach the high school literature. In due time, a generation that knows something of Gibbs as well as of Edison may be expected to support pure science in a manner hitherto lacking in our society. This educational process will afford an essential background to whatever particular measures are taken by either private or public institutions to further scientific advance. In other words, we must work out in a democratic society a public appreciation of pure science, in the place of the support long given it by a more or less aristocratic tradition in Europe.

It is not intended to imply, here, that historical studies should be primarily motivated by practical goals. On the other hand, such contemporary applications as are suggested above in the case of the encouragement of research, are certainly to be welcomed as by-products of historical scholarship.

In view of all these circumstances, it is seriously urged that a number of works be planned to trace the history of the major natural sciences and their technological applications in this country. Not every field would necessarily be undertaken at once. In a few cases, present treatments may be considered adequate; or, again, it may be impossible for some time to find a qualified author who can give the necessary time. It might even prove desirable, first, to experiment modestly with studies in only two or three subjects, especially if the right authors seemed available. But an over-all plan should be worked out looking toward an ultimate treatment of all the chief fields.

In the course of preparing such a plan, various questions concerning subjects, authorship, publication, etc., would inevitably arise. Just what is available on the American story? Should disciplines overlapping the natural and social sciences (geography, anthropology) be included? Would co-authorship be helpful? Should there be a final volume of synthesis? Ought there to be a formal series, brought out in uniform manner by a single publisher? It is unnecessary to answer such queries in advance of actual planning.

A word should be added, however, as to the general standards which should be approximated in the history of any given science. This should ordinarily cover a considerable part of the nation's past (let us say, at least a century), and of the nation's territory. Studies of a more limited scope might well have special values, but would partake of the nature of monographs and would not fully meet the purpose here in view. An adequate history would be interpretive as well as factual. It ought not to bog down in biographical details—a tendency still characteristic of much writing on the history of science—and would in general exhibit the forest as well as the trees. The history of thought should be treated, as well as that of institutions. The story should be presented against both the social and the intellectual background of a given time and place. And, as far as possible within limits imposed by the nature of the materials, the treatment should be intelligible to the serious lay reader.

In conclusion, one very natural objection to these suggestions may be anticipated. It is sometimes held that books should not be planned in series; should not be made to order. One should rather wait for inspiration to strike—laissez faire. No doubt the product of an individual's spontaneous enthusiasm is apt—other things being equal—to be superior to one solicited by a planning board. But there may be times when individuals possessing some potential enthusiasm require encouragement, or need to have their interests correlated with those of similar colleagues, and then a planning group may be of real service. Presumably the latter would never urge an author to undertake a work if he had not already displayed some inclination in that direction. At any rate, in the present instance spontaneous individual interest has failed to produce —decade after decade—the needed works. One may conclude, therefore, that a laissez faire procedure has proved inadequate and that a planned historical program is in order.

XVI

The Interplay
of Social and Internal Factors
in Modern Medicine:

An Historical Analysis *

The simplest classification of the factors involved in the history of a science is that which relates these, first, to the surrounding cultural environment and, second, to the "internal logic" of the science itself. This distinction is not an absolute one [1] but is useful for most purposes, provided that the two categories are broken down into meaningful components. "Cultural environment," for example, includes the technologic, social, and philosophic backgrounds. It also involves professional and institutional circumstances, and independent developments in other sciences. Pertaining to internal logic, in contrast, are the assumptions and objectives of scientists, their approaches (questions asked of Nature), methods employed (logical, and technical), foci of interest, necessary sequences in discovery, evolving ideas, and so on. Also internal to the science is the role of individual genius, in so far as this is deemed a distinct influence in a given field.

So defined, a great part of the first category (environmen-

* Reprinted from *Centaurus*, 1953: 3: 107–125—by permission.
[1] E.g., "foci of interest" are here listed as relating to internal logic, but in certain cases these may be the result of environmental circumstances.

tal) relates to the "social history" of science; and a major portion of the second (internal) category to "the history of scientific thought." But one cannot entirely equate these concepts; for example, the role of a particular, applied technique is an internal one and yet may have little or no influence on scientific thought.

It was usual, during the nineteenth century, to write the history of science largely in terms of the internal aspects. Although some attention was accorded to professional circumstances and to philosophic backgrounds, little heed was given to the intricacies of the total social *milieu*. This oversight or indifference was carried so far, at least in the case of the medical sciences, as almost to imply that these developed within a social vacuum. In order to correct this tendency, much attention has been devoted during recent decades to the "social relations" or the "social history" of science;[2] but this effort has in turn been carried to extremes. One would gather, from some current works, that the development of the sciences was little more than a function of the general cultural environment.[3]

It is not the present purpose to linger with either of these extreme interpretations, although each has its significance for historiography. The view here taken is, rather, that the history of science can be understood only in terms of a

[2] Sufficient literature has appeared on this theme, and on the "sociology of knowledge," as to elicit analyses and bibliographies. For the European literature, see, for example, Robert Merton, *The Sociology of Knowledge*, ISIS, Vol. 27 (Nov., 1937), 493 ff. For the more recent literature, there are a number of bibliographies in English; e.g., M. C. Leikind, *The Social Impact of Science* (Government Printing Office, Washington, D.C., 1945).

[3] It is, of course, entirely justifiable to present the history of scientific developments primarily in relation to the surrounding culture, as in Merle Curti's able work *The Growth of American Thought* (New York, 1943). But there is always some danger of misinterpretation, unless the limitations of this frame of reference are clearly stated; see, e.g., the author's review of this study in the *American Historical Review*, 49 (July, 1944), 732 ff.

constant interplay between internal logic and environment. The omission or even the relative neglect of either of these—however helpful for immediate analysis—will distort any final picture. One may hold, no doubt, that the internal story of a science is of primary concern, in that this is the most distinctive aspect of its history. It is this which makes biology, biology, and not just an indistinguishable thread in a larger pattern. Yet even this statement may be misleading, if it involves emphases not fully justified by the evidence. Much attention, certainly, should be given to the more potent influences to which a science is subjected; and these are not necessarily the most distinctive ones.

The analysis of modern medical history which follows is intended to present—to bring out, as it were—the interplay in that particular field between environmental and internal developments. The sequence employed is a topical rather than a chronologic one, and an attempt is made to be reasonably comprehensive within the limits set by necessary brevity.

One may recall, to begin with, the influence exerted by the European cultural environment as a whole. During the early modern era, pervasive cultural changes—to which science was continuously related as both cause and effect—stimulated and transformed various aspects of "natural philosophy." Medicine [4] then shared with other sciences (as now recognized) the benefits which resulted from certain trends in European life—from trade expansion, the rise of the middle class, the revival of Greek science, new intellectual outlooks, and so on. One need not here review all aspects of the sociology of

[4] "Medicine" is used throughout here in a broad sense, to include medical practice and institutions, the public health, etc., as well as "the medical sciences."

knowledge, or the varied implications of new perspectives, in order to recall the advantages which society gradually extended to science during this epoch. Certain it is that, by 1750, scientific activities were carried on within a social and intellectual setting which was far more conducive to discovery than had been that of the Middle Ages. And it need hardly be added that scientists, taking advantage of this, had by 1750 achieved remarkable results in both basic and applied investigations.

Yet the rate of advance varied widely in different fields. If one accepts the use of quantitative methods as a measure of progress, for example, it is clear that dynamics had reached a level by 1650 which chemistry did not attain until after 1775, and which clinical medicine did not even approach until after 1825. This means that, at any given time between these dates, different sciences were operating on different levels of method and of achievement, despite the fact that all were immersed in a common cultural environment. *A priori,* such contrasts could be ascribed to one or both of the following circumstances: (1) differences in the relationships between the common environment and one science, as compared to another, and (2) differences in the respective natures or internal logic of the various sciences as such.

In the case of medicine, the first theme noted above was of unusual significance. It will be recalled that, despite conditions relatively favorable for science by 1750, there was—from the modern viewpoint—still much to be desired in this connection. It is true that universities were maintained with the help of church, state, and private endowments, and that professors in certain of these institutions were encouraged to pursue original work. But there was little or no direct, financial aid for research in itself. The very establishment of scientific academies, which provided moral support, limited publication facilities, and a few terminal awards, was itself evidence of the inadequacies of the older institutions so far as science was concerned. Few outstanding scientists taught in the universities, and the recruiting of future investigators was anything but systematic.

No doubt the rather casual manner in which research was then supported was more effective than it could be today. The prevailing arrangements were fairly well adapted to the needs of the contemporary physical sciences, since most of the latter were still in a relatively simple stage of development. Research procedures were not complex, technical facilities were neither rich nor rare, and little specialized training was required of investigators. Under these circumstances professors could manage reasonably well without "outside aid," and self-trained amateurs could and did do outstanding work.

The adjustment of medicine to the cultural environment,[5] however, was less satisfactory. Maladjustment here resulted, in part, from a lack of *rapport* between medical science and the society of which it was a part. Unlike the physical or the general biologic sciences, medicine dealt directly with the most vital interests of mankind—with birth and death—and out of this situation arose a whole series of peculiar difficulties. Most obvious, first, was the manner in which the human body (as basic subject matter) was hedged about by all sorts of moral taboos. Physical scientists could do as they pleased with test tubes and pendulums, but physicians must not experiment with living men except within very narrow limits. Popular opposition to the dissection of dead bodies lingered into the nineteenth century, and some abhorrence of autopsies and even of animal experimentation persists to this day.

Physicians could, of course, learn much about disease by a

[5] It should be emphasized that "environment" is also used here in a broad sense. It refers not only to such changing elements as are suggested by terms like "the Enlightenment" or "the romantic era," but also to the whole complex of attitudes, traditions, institutions etc., which were inherited from the past.

passive observation of the sick and by some cautious experiments in treatment. But sound generalizations must be based on many cases, and the traditional "solo" form of medical practice did not enable a physician to see more than a small number of patients. What was needed was an institution in which large numbers of cases could be studied; that is, the hospital. But hospitals had been founded chiefly for humane rather than for scientific ends, and it was not until the nineteenth century that many of them were so organized as to be available for systematic investigations.

If a medical man surmounted the obstacles noted, moreover, he faced still another difficulty inherent in what Roger Bacon once called "the nobility" of his materials. This was the fact that physicians were under constant pressure to get results quickly. This was not usually the case with physical scientists, because the latter's findings were rarely of vital concern to the public. Hence physicists, even though seeking "useful knowledge," could suspend judgment and proceed with due caution. But death would not wait, and so men desired that physicians reach conclusions without benefit of real verification. The insistent need for curing illness had been present throughout the centuries, when the state of medical knowledge was such—we can now see—that it could not possibly meet this demand. Yet the attempt had to be made and, what is more, men ever wished to believe that it had at last been successful. Such wishful thinking constantly encouraged guess-work, unverified speculation, or sheer dogmatism in medical thought.

In addition to the difficulties imposed on medical science by moral or other human considerations, there were further obstacles inherent in the European professional tradition. In the case of physical science, there was no large and ancient guild whose organization or vested interests might retard an effective pursuit of new science. It was far otherwise in medicine. Consider, for example, the diverse manner in which the lack of financial aid for research affected the two fields in the United States. In medicine, by guild tradition in this country, there were rarely any "full-time" professors in medical faculties before 1890. Within the universities, professors of physical science could give all their time to teaching and investigation; but medical instructors were selected from among the best known—and therefore the busiest—practitioners. Such men could pursue original work in their spare moments, as could any self-patron; but the truth was that they had very few moments to spare when lives might be at stake. Cynics may add that professional income was also at stake, but this was not the whole story. Even the wealthy practitioner who was unmoved by humane considerations, and who need never worry about "that damned guinea," found it wise to seek a large practice for the sake of prestige.

In other words, the traditions of the medical guild antedated modern research and only slowly adapted themselves to it. Hence even the more original physicians rarely devoted much time to medical science, giving themselves rather to the related art of medical practice. Comte summed up the situation, early in the nineteenth century, in observing that the prospects for medical science were as dim as they would have been in astronomy, if all research in *that* science had been left to the sea captains.[6]

One may conclude that, although medical science shared in advantages enjoyed by science at large, it also was handicapped by certain unsatisfactory relationships with the cultural environment. Since this lack of *rapport* was more or less

[6] Auguste Comte, *Cours de Philosophie Positive*, III (Paris, 1908; first ed., 1830), 148 ff. Comte, moreover, was doubtless thinking of the European situation, which was not so extreme as that in the United States.

peculiar to medicine, much of the relative lag in this field between 1600 and 1800 may be ascribed to it. But the slow pace of medical progress may also be blamed in part on the other major factor; that is, on the internal nature and logic of medical science as such.

In the first place, biologic phenomena in general—above the level of simple description—were in a sense more complex than were the physical. This was apparently not fully realized in the seventeenth century when, encouraged by the success of dynamics and influenced by the concept of the "animal machine," there was no little enthusiasm for an experimental and quantitative study of the bodies of men and animals. But although the first results were encouraging, as in the discovery of the circulation of the blood, the iatrophysical and iatrochemical schools were largely bogged down by 1700 in a morass of obscure phenomena and conflicting speculations. It was easier in physics than it was in physiology, to isolate problems which could be solved in terms of the knowledge and techniques then available. Hence the zeal of 1700 for quantitative concepts and procedures in medicine, however sound and prophetic in principle, was of small avail at the time.

One may pause here to inquire whether this outcome really involved anything more than just another case of adjusting medicine to the surrounding culture—in this case, to the other sciences. For if the human body was simply an "animal machine"—a matter of controversy between vitalists and materialists—then medicine just called for the application of physical science to this body. And, in that case, medical sciences could only be expected to advance in the wake of the physical.

That there was some truth in this will hardly be denied. Biophysics presupposes an adequate physics, biochemistry an adequate chemistry. But this truism was not so applicable to the medicine of 1700–1850 as it is to that of the present time. This is because much of the significant research of the earlier period was done in pathologic anatomy and related clinical problems, and these fields made little use of either chemistry or physics. Indeed, they usually involved only simple observation, without benefit of the experimental and quantitative methods already taken for granted in the physical disciplines.

In other words, a great part of medical research prior to 1850 was still in the descriptive stage, even as was that in other biologic sciences. But although botanic and zoologic taxonomy presented real difficulties, these were relatively simple in comparison with the complexities and confusions associated with the taxonomic stage of medical developments. It is when one considers this phase of the story that he becomes more aware of problems inherent in medicine as such. As certain of these problems emerged, solutions were attempted along the lines of an internal logic but within limits set—at times—by external circumstance.

Medical thought was in a confused state during the eighteenth century. There was some enthusiasm for Baconian induction in general, and for the Greek clinical tradition in particular. But the Greek heritage also involved a theoretic, generalized pathology which could be neither proved nor disproved by the knowledge and procedures then available. Learned physicians felt it necessary to defend this "rational" pathologic theory, along with more tangible elements in medical knowledge, against the scepticism of the "mere empirics"—a controversy which had likewise been inherited from classical times.[7]

[7] Galen's comments, e.g., are given in A. J. Brock, *Greek Medicine* (London, 1929), 130 ff. On the eighteenth-century form of the controversy, see R. H. Shryock, *Development of Modern Medicine* (London, 1948), Chapter 2.

The rationalists repeated the ancient query: what basic, bodily condition or conditions are involved in illness? They also, in most cases, echoed one of the chief Greek replies; namely, that illness was a condition in which the body fluids or humors (blood, bile, etc.) were impure or out of balance. Once accepted, this theory led logically to a therapy of bleeding and other depletion procedures, intended to eliminate impurities or to restore balance in the "general state of the system." Names had long been given to the more obvious "clinical pictures" (smallpox, great pox, etc.), but there was little interest in disease identification. Since it was the state of the body which the physician treated, and as this seemed much the same in each stage of illness regardless of any names employed, who bother about any exact diagnosis? [8]

This view is not in itself to be lightly dismissed, as has been the wont of medical critics during the past century. It involved some shrewd insights or at least inspired guesses; indeed, it may present us with one of the basic alternatives in outlook to which pathology will from time to time return. But the point here is that the ancient, humoral pathology, as still accepted in the 1700's, was both vague and unconfirmed. Professional discussions of its validity, or of that of opposing theories,[9] were reminiscent of the doctrinal disputes of an earlier scholasticism; rather than of an effort to verify in the manner already established in the physical sciences.

It is true that some physicians defended the speculative pathologies by appealing to the clinical evidence. It was said,

[8] Knud Faber has noted the expression of this view which is found in the concluding statements of the Hippocratic text on *Prognostics;* see his *Thomas Sydenham, der englische Hippocrates u. die Krankheitsbegriffe der Renaissance,* Münchener Med. Wochenscrift, no. 1 (1932), 29.

[9] Somewhat analogous to the humoral tradition was that of the rival tension and laxity (*strictum et laxum*) pathology, which usually related to assumed conditions in the solid parts (solidism) of the nervous or vascular systems. Both these traditions involved speculative, generalized pathology.

or at least implied, that if good results followed upon the application of these theories, then the theories themselves must be sound. Viewed simply in terms of the internal logic— that is, reasoning as one could have done *if* medicine had operated in a social vacuum—the absurdity of this reasoning would have been apparent. *Post hoc, ergo propter hoc* has always been an easy target for those exposing logical fallacies. But the fact is that medicine moved in the rather dense atmosphere of human hopes and fears already noted. Men wished for obvious reasons to believe that medical theories were sound, and under these circumstances were not too critical of the means employed for verification.

There was long no escape from pathologic speculation (with its unhappy encouragement of heroic practice) other than a resort to more or less "crude empiricism." But the empirics, also, had labored long and to no great avail. Scornful of speculation and claiming to be the true Baconians, they sought by unsystematic trial-and-error to discover means of amelioration, prevention, or cure. Even if one assumes that most drugs then known had no rational background—which was not necessarily true—the cumulative achievements of empiricists were hardly impressive. These consisted, apart from the precepts of personal hygiene, of some helpful but dangerous and superficial surgery, and of awesome but largely useless pharmacopoeias. At best, a few drugs of ameliorative value and (by 1700) two actual specifics were known—mercury against syphilis, and cinchona against malaria. And about 1721 the first empirical achievement in preventive medicine—smallpox inoculation—was introduced.[10] Limited as these achievements were, the record was rather impressive when compared with that of the so-called rational school. Yet the latter was correct in its basic assumption that in medicine,

[10] Unless one also includes the use of citrus juice against scurvy in this category—dates here are difficult to determine.

as in all sciences, progress based on principles would be more rapid than that based on blind trial-and-error.

What could these principles be? Since the purpose of physicians was to lessen illness, one would have expected *a priori* that it would be helpful to understand the essential nature of illness; and, if this was a state of the humors, to discover what factors caused this condition. For if causal factors were known, one could then seek rationally for means of avoiding or overcoming them. Most physicians, prior to 1800, had the vaguest notions on this score. They spoke, as had the Greeks, of unhygienic habits, of heredity, of poisons in airs and waters, of contagion, and of what now would be termed psychosomatic influences. A few were even convinced that infections could be traced to minute "insects" or animalculae. But these explanations were rarely verified in any exact manner.

As long as one general state of the body was assumed to underlie all illness, indeed, there was no great interest in causal factors (etiology) except in relation to prevention. For since illness was viewed as basically of the same nature in all cases, physicians focused their attention on this condition. What had originally caused the biliousness, the dropsy, or the fever, was not so important as was the question of how one dealt with such a condition once it had appeared. After all, it was for this curative function that physicians were desired in society. Here one encounters again a limiting social circumstance. Physicians did write at times on preventive hygiene, but laymen usually felt that this was a matter of folklore or common sense. By tradition—and this is still all too true—physicians were called in only to treat acute illness. And at that stage, etiology seemed to the humoralists to be largely an academic matter.

There was, however, another Greek tradition which taught a doctrine essentially different from that of humoralism. The so-called school of Cnidos had held that there was no one pathologic state common to all illness. Rather were there many distinct diseases; from which it followed that there were many distinct causal factors—some or all of them specific for particular diseases. Means of prevention, cures, and prognoses were also likely to be of a specific nature. From this viewpoint, the first purpose of physicians was to discover these different diseases; for one could hardly seek the prevention or cure of a particular disease until this entity was itself identified.

From the time of Galen until the sixteenth century the humoralist tradition dominated medicine, while the Cnidian was recessive. Just why a few physicians then revived emphasis on the latter is not clear. Increasing knowledge of non-Galenic, Greek medical literature may have had something to do with it. There were always clinical phenomena, of course, which suggested differences in types of illness; and it is conceivable that a renewed attention to these differences resulted from a slow but pervasive improvement of observation in general. More definitely, it has been suggested that the discovery of a remedy which was helpful against *only one* type of illness, implied that this "clinical picture" must be distinct from all others. The most striking instance here was the discovery that cinchona bark was a specific for a certain type of fever (malaria), which made a deep impression on physicians during the seventeenth century.[11]

Whatever the explanations, the doctrine of specificity was clearly revived and emphasized during the latter part of that century. The most sweeping presentation was that of the English clinician Sydenham, who held that diseases were as real and diverse as were species of plants and animals. Each disease entity had its own causes, its own natural history, and

[11] Knud Faber, *op. cit.*

even—if these only could be found—its own cures.[12] The
optimism implicit in this outlook has not always been fully
appreciated, but it must thereafter have had an increasingly
stimulating impact upon medical thought. Instead of continued dependence on the shopworn and static doctrines of
humoralism, those who accepted the concept of specificity
could envisage new and promising discoveries all along the
advancing front of medicine.

This optimism, although it may have originated in Greek
ideas and was, in any case, internal to medical thinking, was
encouraged because it harmonized with—and perhaps contributed to—the general optimism of the Enlightenment era.
More than this, and here again is the interplay between
internal logic and cultural environment, the subsequent
triumphs of the specificity concept were made possible in part
by developments outside of medicine—especially by independent advances in other sciences.

This is not to claim that it was easy at first to identify
specific diseases, to say nothing of finding specific cures for
the same. It was difficult even to determine what criteria of
identification could be employed. Sydenham and his successors defined disease entities largely by symptoms—a procedure which had always been vaguely followed in giving
names to different patterns of illness. But when attempts were
made to do this in a more systematic and exact manner, the
effort bogged down in the multiplicity of symptoms and their
combinations. The nosology texts of the later 1700's listed and
classified almost two thousand so-called diseases, but these
lists involved little more than names for that number of
symptom combinations. So confusing did this situation become that some medical leaders maintained, or returned to,

---

[12] Benjamin Rush, (ed.), *Works of Thomas Sydenham* . . . (Philadelphia, 1809), xxiv ff.

the view that there was only one underlying pathologic state in all forms of illness.[13]

Neither an endless list of names, on the one hand, nor pathologic speculation on the other, could ever have stimulated much further research. The physician who believed there was only one underlying pathology—with some one basic treatment deduced therefrom—already knew all the answers. Why bother with more investigations? No matter how encouraging the cultural environment, medical progress would have been almost impossible as long as these internal convictions had been maintained.

Fortunately, the energy imparted by the concept of specificity carried medicine over this barrier of nosographical confusion. During the very era when symptoms alone were proving to be inadequate for disease identification, a second criterion emerged from medical research. The clue to this was found in the study of human anatomy, which had first been pursued in classical Alexandria, was undertaken once more in late medieval Europe, and was finally brought to a flourishing state during the Italian Renaissance. As research in normal anatomy expanded, it led by an almost inevitable, internal logic to a study of morbid anatomy as well.

The view that there was a relationship between structural changes in the body and illness was first expressed in classical Alexandria, but was thereafter largely lost to sight during the long dominance of generalized humoralism. Perhaps the possibilities were never entirely forgotten in the more obvious instances; for example, it was suggested even in medieval autopsies that crude obstructions might occasion illness. But normal, gross anatomy had first to be carefully investigated

---

[13] E.g., Dr. Benjamin Rush of Philadelphia announced about 1800, as a "new" theory, that there was only one pathologic state. He was then hailed by many as having brought order out of the chaos of the nosologies. A long poem to this effect is preserved in his papers in that city.

(1500–1750) before its implications for morbid anatomy could be demonstrated.

It has recently been pointed out by Temkin that surgeons played a significant role in drawing attention to the relationships between structural changes and disease. Surgeons, in the nature of the case, had always dealt with structural conditions. They necessarily "had to rely on physical signs in their diagnosis and had to correlate the clinical picture to structural changes." These procedures were followed more effectively as surgery improved, once it was provided with a sound anatomical basis. It is true that surgeons usually dealt with injuries on the surface, rather than with those hidden within the body (lesions); but all that was needed in order to provide a complete structural pathology, was to transfer surgical attitudes *re* superficial injuries to internal injuries as well.

This transfer was delayed by lack of professional contacts between European surgeons and physicians—an environmental factor—but traditional barriers between the two guilds were partly overcome in certain countries even before 1750. As a result, some leading physicians were already familiar with surgical outlooks at that time. There is contemporary testimony by internists that it was this familiarity which finally encouraged them to think in terms of a structural pathology. The latter concept was first systematically presented in the work of Morgagni (1761), who was not a surgeon; but it was ignored for decades thereafter by most internists. Not until surgeons and physicians were brought into close association in the Paris school of about 1800, did the localized, structural pathology become dominant.[14]

It was realized, after this time, that a correlation of *ante*

[14] Owsei Temkin, *The Role of Surgery in the Rise of Modern Medical Thought*, Bulletin of the History of Medicine, 25 (May–June, 1951), 248 ff.

mortem symptoms with *post mortem* pathologic data could reveal disease patterns which were more clear-cut and distinctive than were those composed of symptoms alone. A great impetus was thereby given, not only to autopsy studies, but also to the improvement of clinical investigations. As has often been said, physicians prior to 1800 *observed* their patients; thereafter, they began to *examine* them. The introduction of improved research methods in clinical medicine subsequently owed much to the cultural environment, in terms of mathematics and physics; as when the former made statistics available, and the latter (in association with technology) produced microscopes and other 'scopes which followed. But even more basic was the internal transformation wrought when physicians came to *look* for localized pathology; as is indicated by the fact that their first new instruments of observation (the hand, in percussion, and the stethoscope) were developed empirically without aid from contemporary physics or technology.

Between 1800 and 1850, rapid progress was made in the identification of many diseases as still generally recognized, in terms of the correlation of clinical and pathologic data. In the place of the old humoral theories, or even of vague symptomatic notions like "inflammation of the chest" or "peri-pneumonia," there appeared such relatively specific concepts as "pneumonia" and "bronchitis." In the place of confused, symptomatic notions of various "fevers" (intermittent, continuous, remittent, etc.), there emerged the concepts of typhus, typhoid, malaria, and the like.[15]

In consequence medical research was ready, by about 1850, to undertake the next step which Sydenham had long before envisaged; that is, to seek out the causal factors and cures of these now-identified diseases. In so doing, moreover, it was

[15] The evolution of these concepts can be traced by comparing old "bills of mortality" with the later lists of "causes of death."

aided by improved methods which could not have been employed prior to identification. Thus the microscope (an instrument known long before this) could not have been used in a search for specific pathogenic organisms until the diseases to which these were related were clearly recognized. Pasteur could never have found organisms which were causal factors in such vaguely-conceived conditions as "biliousness," or "inflammation of the chest." In like manner, Louis could never have introduced clinical statistics as a check on therapeutic procedures, until he had first known the diseases with which he was dealing.

Up to this point, medical opinion had varied on the somewhat metaphysical question concerning the ultimate nature of diseases. Were they, as Sydenham held, objective entities—even as plant or animal species? Were diseases something real and outside of men, which invaded their bodies—a notion reminiscent of ancient, demoniac lore? There was considerable resistance to this "ontologic" concept, even among pathologists of the later nineteenth century, who tended to think of disease in a nominalistic manner as simply a form of bodily response to certain stimuli. Instead of viewing this response as involving the bodily "system" as a whole, however, they now thought of response in particular parts—in organs, tissues, or cells, depending on the historic stage of research involved.

When, after 1870, specific, pathogenic micro-organisms were discovered, bacteriologists at first viewed them as solely responsible for the related infections. And as long as typhoid bacilli were thought of as *the* cause of typhoid fever, it was easy to think of this disease as an entity—incarnate in the bacilli, so to speak, and loose in the community. Subsequent developments in immunology and other fields reduced the pathogenic organisms to the status of merely "*a* causal factor," however, and the concept of disease as bodily response has again become dominant. All of this relates in part to internal developments in medicine, but it was also conditioned by the philosophic perspectives of medical scientists. Hence one should turn again, at this point, to the interaction of the internal developments with the surrounding cultural environment of the nineteenth century.

Each of the major philosophic outlooks of the eighteenth and nineteenth centuries had its implications for medical thought, despite the long-run trend toward divorcing modern science from metaphysics. Both philosophic empiricism and materialism encouraged scientific research, as did the subsequent development of Comte's positivism. The relationship between these "schools" and medical thought was at times quite definite, as when the *idéologues* of Paris encouraged, about 1800, the very program of objective clinical and pathologic research which has been mentioned.[16] The influence exerted by German idealism after 1815 was more complex and obscure. There is no doubt that the *Naturphilosophie* encouraged some return to grandiose speculation in pathology and related fields, especially in Germany between that date and about 1840. But there were only minor responses to this in certain other Western countries, as in the United States; and, in any case, the more extreme versions of this outlook were abandoned even in Germany thereafter. Some of the more subtle implications of the *Naturphilosophie*, moreover, may actually have had value for the great flowering of German research which then ensued.[17]

[16] George Rosen, *The Philosophy of Ideology and the Emergence of Modern Medicine in France*, Bulletin of the History of Medicine, 20 (July, 1946), 328 ff.

[17] See, e.g., Walter Pagel, *The Speculative Basis of Modern Pathology. Jahn, Virchow and the Philosophy of Pathology*, Bulletin of the History of Medicine, 18 (June, 1945) 1 ff.

More apparent than the influence of philosophy, was that exerted by social conditions and outlooks upon medicine during the nineteenth century. Certain aspects of this were favorable: the increase of wealth and of urban population resulting from the industrial revolution eventually benefited scientific institutions in many obvious ways. More specifically, the growth of cities, cheaper printing, and improved transportation facilitated the development of medical societies, research institutes, libraries, publications, and the like. Most important for medicine was the evolution of the large hospital —a product of social pressures—from a custodial institution into the type of research center needed for the clinical and pathologic studies of the times.

It need hardly be added that the striking progress made in other natural sciences during the nineteenth century proved of major advantage to medicine. This story is too well known to need repetition here; but it may be noted again that the impact of the other sciences did not become obvious until after about 1850. This was not only because progress in these became more rapid thereafter but also because medicine itself had first to go through the taxonomic and other stages mentioned, before it could fully avail itself of contributions from related fields.

On the other hand, there were certain aspects of social change which were less favorable for medicine. Or, to be more exact, the interplay between certain aspects of internal medical developments and a changing society was less favorable. Consider, for example, the social reactions of 1825–1875 to the expanding program of clinical and pathologic research. As already noted, it is difficult to see how basic progress in medicine could ever have been achieved except along this line. Yet the program was centered for more than fifty years on the identification of diseases, rather than on their prevention or cure. Research men were so preoccupied with this "pure" research, which had no immediate prospect of utility, that they lost interest in therapy. Moreover, their more critical temper led them to discard the older remedies, at a time when there was as yet little with which to replace them. A spirit of "medical nihilism" pervaded the best centers.

In so far as this nihilism became known to the public, it was not calculated to inspire confidence in medical practice. There is indeed evidence that this period, which we can now see was of great promise in medicine, was one in which the public had the least confidence in regular practice. One of the indications of this was the proliferation of rival medical sects, such as homeopathy, hydrotherapy, "the botanic system" (Thomsonianism), and so on. These sects preserved the old thesis of a single, generalized pathologic state, or of some single scheme of treatment, long after these over-simple formulae had been repudiated in regular medicine. Then they promised the cures which the more candid regular physicians no longer believed possible, and so appealed to a public which was often in dire need of such assurances.[18]

More serious than popular doubts, moreover, was the danger that neither philanthropists nor governments were likely to support a field having little apparent utility. Modern science had early been hailed as a means to acquiring "useful knowledge"; and if this was indeed its major purpose, why assist it when it failed to serve that end?

The answer to this query was not a simple one. Actually, little direct private or governmental aid was extended to pure research in medicine or biology prior to 1860. But in relatively aristocratic countries not yet dominated by industrialism, science continued to benefit from the deference long accorded to learning as such. This can be best observed in the prestige enjoyed by German or other Continental professors, and the

[18] R. H. Shryock, *Quackery and Sectarianism in American Medicine,* The Scalpel, May, 1949.

support extended to them by their respective governments. It even became a matter of pride with some men that their research had no relation to "mere utility."

In relatively democratic countries, where business men became increasingly influential, the middle classes continued to encourage the pursuit of useful knowledge. Conversely, they had little desire to support basic research. This attitude could be observed to some degree in England, but found its extreme expression in the United States, where a "practical" people saw little reason for supporting the "idle curiosity" of pathologists or other pure scientists. It is hardly an exaggeration to say that, for most Americans, the word science connoted simply "applied science" or technology.[19]

It is suggestive that in those countries where science was highly regarded for its own sake, there were notable achievements during the nineteenth century. This can be well observed in medicine, where the preëminence of French and German pathologists was widely recognized. Even more striking was the manner in which the French and Germans dominated bacteriology, as this field emerged after 1875. At the other extreme, again, was the experience of the United States, where—despite individual exceptions—the record in basic medical research was a negligible one. Had the matter been left to this country, it is unlikely that "modern medicine" as we understand it would ever have evolved. At best, the process would have taken a much longer time. Hence we have the paradox that, in pursuing immediately practical goals, the Americans proved in the long run to be a quite impractical people.[20]

[19] R. H. Shryock, *American Indifference to Basic Science During the Nineteenth Century,* Archives Internationales d'Historie des Sciences, No. 5 (Oct., 1948), 50 ff.

[20] Tocqueville, in analyzing this situation in 1835, thought that Americans would have developed basic science if they had lacked European aid. But he cited Chinese civilization as having failed to do this under those circumstances. (*Democracy in America,* New York, 1904, vol. II, 518.) One also thinks of the analogy of the practical Romans.

The fact that technology made rapid progress in the United States might conceivably have led to parallel advances in basic science there. Certainly there are circumstances in which one can observe technology stimulating science, as well as *vice versa*.[21] This was true even in medicine; for example, when knowledge of brewing and fermentation played a role in Pasteur's investigations. But whatever was true in special cases, the American story certainly indicates that applied science and technology *may* be successfully cultivated on a large scale without any major benefit to basic science. It also suggests that an exclusive devotion to applied science may even interfere with, or at least divert attention from, basic science. Americans were quite successful at times in applied medical science, as in the introduction of anesthesia and in other contributions to surgery. Yet these achievements did little, prior to 1900, to stimulate basic research in medicine as a whole.

During the present century, one of the most striking internal trends in medical science has been the partial return to a generalized pathology. Beginning with a limited revival of humoral pathologic concepts (as in immunology and endocrinology), this trend was extended (in terms of nutritional research, psychosomatic studies, and so on) still further in the direction of a generalized pathology. Much of this involved simply the superimposing on structural pathology of more general concepts. But in the recent development of the sulfa-drugs and antibiotics, and more especially of cortisone and ACTH therapy, a more complete return to the outlook of a generalized, systemic pathology has been suggested. The first reaction seems to have been the thought that if certain

[21] See, e.g., S. Lilley's interesting analysis of the relationship between technology and the laws of thermodynamics, *Social Aspects of the History of Science,* Archives Internationales d'Historie des Sciences, no. 6 (Jan., 1949), 376 ff.

drugs could "cure" many apparently distinct diseases, all of the latter must really have some underlying pathology in common; i.e., they are not really specific at all.

One notes here, again, what a potent influence pharmacology has apparently exerted at certain key points on the course of medical thought. Just as the discovery of a specific drug in the seventeenth century may have then revived the idea of disease specificity, so now the discovery of non-specific drugs may revive the concept of non-specific disease processes. To some contemporary medical men, the latter outlook seems "an entirely new concept"; which is natural enough in case their perspective is limited to the last hundred years.[22] The historical background, however, provides protection against such extreme awe for the accomplishments of our own generation.

The clinical evidence, as well as the historical, also suggests caution here. Apparently, in the case of acute infections, the new drugs may remove or suppress the symptoms without eliminating the disease process. This implies that the concept of specificity will continue to be useful in this area, even though there will be no such exclusive dependence on it as was the case only a generation ago. The results of cortisone and ACTH therapy in chronic disease have been more encouraging, even though actual cures have been rarely if ever involved; but it may be that observations have not yet been sufficiently prolonged to be certain of the conclusions.

Of course, if a drug which is literally a "cure-all" is ever

[22] See, e.g., the statements by Dr. J. S. L. Browne of McGill University that: ". . . the symptoms of tuberculosis are the manifestations of the injury inflicted by the tubercle bacilli. But underlying them is the *general* response of the body to damage, *any damage* . . . This philosophical point of view greatly alters our concept of disease . . . And this idea . . . is completely at variance with the older views of scientific medicine." Quoted by George W. Grey, *Cortisone and ACTH*, Scientific American, vol. 182 (March, 1950), 35, 36. Italics are those of the author.

discovered, we would then probably return to the notion of one underlying pathologic state; but no such idyllic prospect looms before us at present. Meantime, the unexpected results of cortisone therapy raise some interesting questions; for example, are we to conceive of a disease as something quite distinct from its symptoms? But, if so, what are the underlying pathologic processes involved, other than merely some sort of internal "symptoms"? The concept of disease, apparently so obvious, actually remains a rather baffling one.

These recent internal trends in medical research have no obvious relationship to the social environment, other than to increase public confidence in medical practice. But much confidence had already been revived by striking progress all along the line in medicine during the past seventy-five years. The social implications or interactions of this general, internal progress were complex. The technical advances which made the public seek medical care, for example, also made that commodity more expensive; so that the more this care was desired, the less people could afford it. Out of this situation, in part, has grown the demand for government health insurance systems. And these systems, in turn, are likely to influence medical research as well as practice, for either good or ill.

The revival of confidence in medicine after 1870 had far-reaching implications, not only for medical care but also for the support of medical research. Outside of English-speaking lands, nearly all medical schools were located in state-supported universities; and ministries of education gradually increased the funds available to these schools as well as to other scientific faculties. In order to initiate new specialized programs, moreover, special research institutes were set up for outstanding scientists—those established for Pasteur, Ehrlich, and Koch come readily to mind. Some of these were state-supported, others were given private endowments; some were autonomous institutions, others became units within universities.

In English-speaking countries the very emphasis upon the practical, which had hitherto inhibited basic investigations, now encouraged them—once it became clear that these really promised utility of a new order. This was particularly fortunate because Britain and the United States were wealthy nations, in an age when research was becoming ever more expensive. In the United States before 1900, medicine had played the role of a neglected Cinderella; but thereafter it became the chief beneficiary of great private foundations. Beginning with the 1920's in Britain, and the '30's in the States, medicine—as well as other sciences—also received increasing support from governmental sources.[23]

The recent trend toward state aid, which may be interpreted as a reaction against earlier *laissez-faire* attitudes toward science, was carried much further in fascist and communist societies. In the latter, state support of medical and other scientific research has been accompanied by state control; and in the Western countries fear of such control has now dramatized the whole theme of the relations between science and society.[24]

One may close the discussion with this brief note on recent developments, which are obviously of great significance. Both the internal developments within medicine, and social transformations in its environment, now proceed at an accelerated pace. The interplay between the two is as inevitable now as in times past, but the actual components and results of the process are changing rapidly.

[23] R. H. Shryock, *American Medical Research: Past and Present* (New York, 1947), Chapts. 4, 8.
[24] *Cf.* J. D. Bernal, *Social Function of Science* (New York, 1939), Chapt. 1; and M. Polanyi, *The Contempt of Freedom: The Russian Experiment and After* (London, 1940).

Index

333

Medicine in America
Historical Essays

by Richard Harrison Shryock

designer: Cecilie Smith
typesetter: Kingsport Press, Inc.
typefaces: Fairfield (text) and Deepdene (display)
printer: Kingsport Press, Inc.
paper: Warren's Olde Style
binder: Kingsport Press, Inc.
cover material: Holliston Roxite